# The Guide to Breast Reconstruction

Step-by-step from Mastectomy
through Reconstruction

# Patricia O'Grady

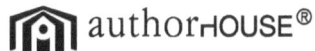
authorHOUSE®

*AuthorHouse™ LLC*
*1663 Liberty Drive*
*Bloomington, IN 47403*
*www.authorhouse.com*
*Phone: 1-800-839-8640*

*Published by AuthorHouse 02/21/2014*

*ISBN: 978-1-4918-6693-1 (sc)*
*ISBN: 978-1-4918-6690-0 (hc)*
*ISBN: 978-1-4918-6692-4 (e)*

*Library of Congress Control Number: 2014903309*

*Special thanks to Dwayne Colborn for his modification of the cover picture.*

*Any people depicted in stock imagery provided by Thinkstock are models, and such images are being used for illustrative purposes only.*
*Certain stock imagery © Thinkstock.*

*This book is printed on acid-free paper.*

*"Some people think having large breasts makes a woman stupid. Actually, it's quite the opposite. A woman having large breasts makes men stupid."*
Rita Rudner


*"Once I overcame breast cancer, I wasn't afraid of anything anymore."*
Melissa Etheridge


*"A woman without breasts is like a bed without pillows."*
Anatole France


*"Breast cancer is scary and no one understands that like another woman who has gone through it too."*
Mindy Sterling


*"Breast cancer is not for sissies."*
Suzanne Somers


*"My breast cancer scare changed my life. I'm grateful for every new, healthy day I have. It has helped me prioritize my life."*
Olivia Newton-John


*"Breast cancer is the disease that, for a long time, women feared the most. In this country, we're so focused on physical looks. We tie the issue of femininity to physical appearance, and people think primarily of breast cancer that threatens your breasts — though those who have it realize, more significantly, that it threatens your life."*
Fran Visco

*"If only women paid as much attention
to their breasts as men do."*
Patricia O'Grady

*This book is dedicated to Dr. John B. Roach and Kirsty Metcalf.*

*I am eternally grateful for your wise counsel and amazing skills.*

# Table of Contents

# GETTING IT OFF MY CHEST—Introduction

There are many books available on the subject of breast cancer. These cover a variety of topics, including diagnosis, cancer treatments and personal stories about the battle but not many are dedicated exclusively to the subject of breast reconstruction. I remember my consultation, sitting in the plastic surgeon's office feeling totally overwhelmed. My head was swimming with all kinds of thoughts as I tried hard to concentrate and actually listen to him, while he carefully explained my options and the lengthy process. I realize now that I probably only heard and maintained half of the things he had said to me that day. As I went through my own personal journey, I realized that I needed more information about the road ahead. I wished for a step-by-step guide to help me through the process, preferably written by someone who had compassion and insight. I had no use for medical terms that I didn't fully understand, written by someone quoting medical journals who had never actually experienced what I would be undertaking. I wanted to hear words from a woman who was uniquely qualified to discuss the subject because she had actually completed what I was just beginning. There are two sides to this story: the doctor telling you what you can expect and the patient telling you what she actually experienced not only physically but mentally, and emotionally. This entire process requires both you and your doctor to work together as a team. While he does the technical work of the surgeries, it's up to you to follow all your post-op instructions so that you will achieve the best results.

I always seemed to have questions that I would forget to ask during my doctor's visits. I take much comfort in knowing that I was truly blessed with a wonderful doctor and staff. They made it clear I could call their office anytime I had a question, but they couldn't offer me a 24-hour hotline. On those sleepless nights, I did what most people do nowadays: I searched the Internet seeking answers. What I discovered is that the web seems to have a wealth of misinformation, at least on this particular subject, which only increased my anxiety, fears and concerns. I have come to the conclusion that people seem to post when they have had a negative experience, but they rarely post when they've had a positive one. You have to learn to ignore everything that is not motivating you, not inspiring you and not allowing you to move forward, because it's utterly useless.

I felt obligated to write this book to provide practical guidance for my fellow travelers. As I went through each surgery and recovery, I told myself that once my breast reconstruction was complete, I would open the next chapter in my own life and pen this book. It is a comfortable medium and forum that will allow me to not only share my recent experience with others; it will also give me the satisfaction of knowing that I have helped other women, even if only in some small way.

On some level, this is a challenging proposition because, even though my story has a wonderful end, I know many victims of this insidious disease may not be as fortunate. I honor those who have lost their battle and succumbed to breast cancer. I salute my fellow survivors, and I encourage and support those who choose to have breast reconstruction.

# MY BREAST CANCER STORY

Before I take you through all of the steps of breast reconstruction, I want to give you a *very* brief summary of my own personal breast cancer diagnosis and treatment. I don't want this book to be about ME; I want this book to be about YOU! During the course of this book, I will walk you through my experience, telling you my thoughts and feelings so you know what I felt not only physically but emotionally.

Having breast cancer was my destiny; there was really no way around it. Although I have always thought of myself as being a positive thinker, I knew being positive could not change what was in my gene pool. I unknowingly put myself at greater risk by taking estrogen hormone replacement drugs after having a total hysterectomy at the age of 27. I was prescribed and took Premarin for 23 years. The doctor immediately ordered me to stop taking it when I was diagnosed with breast cancer—obviously a little too late.

I guess, for me, it wasn't *if* I would ever get breast cancer; it was more like *when* I would get it. On some level, I thought of myself as a walking time bomb, and I knew the detonation could happen at any time. Ever since I was a teenager, I had known that at some point in my life, I would be facing this scary disease because of the deep-seated family history of breast cancer. Two of my aunts passed away from breast cancer when I was a child. My mother had a mastectomy at the young age of 43 due to stage 4 breast cancer, followed by a year of radiation treatments and chemo-therapy. She fought the battle hard and she won; she's a true survivor. She didn't opt for breast reconstruction and has lived the last 33 years wearing a breast form. Although she has always maintained that she has no regrets about not doing breast reconstruction, she has been fully supportive of my decision to do it and went with me to many of my doctor's appointments. I love her for that, because deep down at times during this process, I have felt a little guilty that I was getting new breasts, and she was still wearing her prosthesis.

I fear for my 25-year-old daughter because, unless science can find a way to stop it, her future could very well follow the same exact path. As of this writing, she is scheduled for the genetic BRCA testing and is considering preventive double mastectomies with reconstruction, depending on the results of that testing. That's quite a large burden to carry for a young girl and, sadly, she is just one of many in this position.

I was diligent about having my yearly mammogram. I started at the age of 27 and never missed a year of the crushing routine. Every year, I held my breath wondering if this would be the time the ax would fall. It was always a great relief when they told me all was well. The last three mammograms I had were followed several days later with the dreaded call back. They insisted on doing a digital mammogram, followed by an ultrasound. They told me my breast tissue was extremely dense, which made my mammograms harder to read. They wanted a better look, just to be sure, they said. Each time, I felt slightly panicked, especially because I had noticed tenderness in my left nipple and areola that was increasingly getting worse. I tried to convince myself that this was from natural hormone changes in my body and completely normal. I reported this tenderness, but the doctors didn't seem overly concerned; therefore, I decided I shouldn't worry about it either. During the first two years of callbacks, I got the all-clear after the tests had been completed, which was a great relief. I went on with my daily life and wouldn't even think about my breasts until the following year when I was due for the next routine mammogram. Ironically, even knowing my high-risk situation, I never did the recommended monthly breast self-exams; I just relied on my yearly mammogram, which I'm actually ashamed to admit. I make no excuses for that; I knew better, and I should have done it.

In March 2013, at the age of 50, my time had run out. I was called back for a cone biopsy after the digital mammogram and ultrasound had been completed. I had been diagnosed with invasive ductal carcinoma in my left breast; later I would learn it was already at stage 2. On May 14, 2013 (the very day that actress Angelina Jolie announced that she had undergone a *preventive* double mastectomy), I was on the operating table having a double mastectomy to rid my body of cancer.

My lymph node biopsy came back clean. Chemotherapy was offered as a "just to be sure" scenario, but I made the decision to pass on it. I could handle losing my breasts, but not my long blond hair. I had previously survived cervical cancer, which led to the loss of my uterus, cervix, fallopian tubes and both ovaries. And now, after a double mastectomy, the thought of losing my hair was just too much to bear; I was afraid it would strip me of my last little bit of femininity. Missing all of these female body parts, in a way, made me feel like I was an "it" instead of a female. I have worn my hair long most of my life. A haircut to me consists of a half-inch trim (*note that the hairdresser and I need to have a true understanding of

6

the definition of what a half inch actually is before this trim can begin). My hair has grown to the point where I could actually sit on it. My mane is, in some strange way, part of my identity. Therefore, I have been determined not to part with these golden locks unless, they tell me down the line that my life is on the line.

When I received my diagnosis, I decided to do something a little bold and out of character to change my appearance. I used hair color to place a pink streak in my hair, which I still proudly wear to this day, although over time the meaning of it has changed. Initially, I think I put it in my hair almost to protest what I had ahead of me. Perhaps, in a way, I did it to show my total rebellion against chemotherapy and that I would be keeping my hair. During my surgeries and reconstruction, I wore it to show others what I was going through, because there were times, in certain clothing, when my lack of breasts was obvious. It was a way of giving others an explanation of my situation without having to speak about it and bare my soul. Now I wear it as a reminder of what I have been through, and how lucky I am; it's my own personal badge of honor.

# BREAST DAYS AHEAD—The decisions

You will face a number of confusing choices in your own health care. While the doctors will offer their expert advice, in the end, remember that you are the one who will live with the results of any surgery or treatments. Don't feel that you must make an instant decision overnight as to the course of your treatment. Take a week or two, and really think about all the options that you have been given. This is a life-changing decision, one that will alter your body forever; it's not a decision that you should feel pressured into making overnight.

If you have been offered the choice of having either a lumpectomy or a mastectomy, find out what the final outcomes for you would be; each case has to be considered individually. Before you go under the knife to have one of these surgeries, make an appointment with a plastic surgeon that specializes in breast reconstruction and have a consultation. This will be money well spent because he will be able to give you a clear understanding of your reconstruction options so that you can make an informed choice. Let him guide you in your choices, based on where the cancer is in your breast and the size of it. Obviously, it is easier for him to repair damage before it has happened, go to him before the mastectomy, if possible. You want him to be in the operating room assisting with your mastectomy, or even doing that actual surgery.

This consultation appointment proved to be a lifesaver for me because he not only showed me pictures; he took the time to explain things to me that the oncologist *never* told me. I walked in with the options the oncologist offered me, either a lumpectomy followed by radiation treatments (which I believe I was leaning toward) or a left breast mastectomy. When I left that consultation, I was no longer confused or overwhelmed. I was strong and confident in the decision to have not only a mastectomy but also to have the healthy breast removed as well. Once I made that choice, I never looked back. I'm happy with my decision; for me, it was a no-brainer.

When I walked into this appointment, I honestly didn't even want to be there; in fact, I had almost canceled it that morning. The evening before, I had my first and, I'd like to think, my last emotional meltdown. I had the attitude that I didn't want to do any of it. I was determined to find another way out. I was a smart woman and I could find another solution to this cancer thing. Looking back, I realize now that this was my short period of denial before coming to terms with the fact that I actually had breast cancer, something that would not just go away. There was no magical way out of this; I needed to face it and deal with it, one day at a time. Surprisingly, I left that doctor's visit telling myself that everything was going to be all right.

Learning the real facts about a lumpectomy helped me make my decision to have a double mastectomy. A lumpectomy is the removal of the breast tumor and some of the normal tissue that surrounds it. This is a form of breast-conserving or breast-preservation surgery, which sounded good when it was first presented to me. Technically, a lumpectomy is a partial mastectomy because part of the breast tissue is removed. You must understand that the amount of tissue removed can vary greatly in this kind of surgery, which can dramatically affect the asymmetry between your breasts, the shape of the affected breast and the scarring on it. This may seem like the easier way out, and for some it is, as long as you understand that your breasts will no longer match in size and shape. Virtually all patients who undergo lumpectomy will require some radiation. You should know that having radiation treatments alters your options down the road regarding some of the different kinds of breast reconstruction; so once you make this decision, there may be no turning back. Should you decide to go the route of having a lumpectomy, make sure you have a clear understanding from your surgeon beforehand about how much of your breast may be gone after surgery and what kind of scar you will have.

I was shocked when the plastic surgeon showed me pictures of lumpectomies. This was not what I had pictured in my mind at all. Some of the breasts were so disfigured and horrible. I remember each and every one of these pictures clearly, even a year after seeing them. There were plenty of attractive "before" pictures but no pretty "after" pictures. In some cases, nothing can be done to help these women. I'm quite sure that none of these ladies chose a lumpectomy knowing that permanent disfigurement would be their final result. I previously thought that having a lumpectomy would mean saving my breast. After seeing the outcome of some of these surgeries, I realized I would be saving nothing, and possibly creating something truly hideous that I would have to live with forever. Many of these women end up having the deformed breast removed in the end, so that they can have breast reconstruction. On the other end of it, you will find other women who made the decision to have a lumpectomy, and they are quite happy with their choice; it's all very personal.

No decision is right or wrong; it comes down to what is the right or wrong decision for you.

An added advantage to having a mastectomy is that many patients may not require any chemotherapy or radiation. The need for radiation or chemotherapy is determined by the tumor type, grade and location, the size of the margins, the proximity to the skin and the underlying muscle. Most of the time a woman who is a candidate for a lumpectomy has a very small, low-grade tumor. In these cases, performing a mastectomy alone may be sufficient, along with sentinel node biopsy.

Radiation has progressive, ongoing effects on the breast, which continue indefinitely. After a lumpectomy, there will be contraction of that breast on a progressive basis. In most circumstances, patients who have radiation don't do as well if they have implants because of the skin contraction that occurs as a result of the radiation. Usually, a flap reconstruction will work better or a combination of flap and implant. Keep in mind that irradiated tissue will never be the same. Operating in a field that has been previously irradiated is more difficult because of the changes in the elasticity of skin and alterations in natural tissue planes. Often, the risks for bleeding and infection are elevated. For patients, this means slower healing, increased bruising, and a potential for an increase in wound complications. Some plastic surgeons will refuse to do any surgery if you have had radiation in that particular area due to the reasons above. Search for one that has a lot of experience with operating on irradiated tissue. Keep in mind that if you manage to avoid all the risks associated with radiation, the final results still may not be completely optimal.

From a cosmetic and reconstructive standpoint, it's usually easier to have a simple mastectomy and breast reconstruction. For that matter, it's usually easier to make a completely new set of symmetric breasts than it is to modify the natural breast with reduction, enlargement or lift to match the reconstructed one. The other obvious advantage to this is that removing the healthy breast reduces your risk of breast cancer down the road. My personal thinking is: Why go through this twice when you can do it once and be done with it? I'm hesitant to say I'm cancer-free; I mean, no one can really know that for sure, although I certainly like to think positively. I'm smart enough to know that a double mastectomy doesn't mean I won't ever get cancer again. I know what I had, and I know what I did to get rid of it. It's about well-informed choices and increasing your odds. I know what might happen down the road, but in the end, it's not just about the statistics; it's about the woman and the quality of her life.

After you decide whether or not you will have a lumpectomy or a mastectomy, many other choices still need to be made: single mastectomy, double mastectomy, skin nipple and areola sparing mastectomy, implant, flap procedure, breast size, nipple and areola reconstruction, nipple tattooing, artistic tattoo, radiation and chemo. Fortunately, you don't have to make all of the decisions now. Take it one step at a time. You can decide how far you want to take this when you reach that point. Each option has its pros and cons. Of course, they are all preferable to having no options at all.

I have unending admiration for the women who have lost their breasts to cancer and have chosen not to reconstruct. I think they are just as beautiful as women who've never gone through cancer and those who have gone through it and opted for reconstructive surgery. But after much debate with myself,

I had to choose another path. The decision brought with it a great feeling of liberation once I made it. I felt released from the pressure I was putting on myself to make all the right choices for my future. I pushed away the underling feelings of being judged by others for vainness. I decided that if others considered me to be vain for wanting breasts, then so be it; I could live with that label. Why should I defend my position of wanting to feel beautiful or for the need to feel whole? Remember that you owe no one an explanation for your decision to have fake breasts; this is your body, and this is your choice to make.

I don't need to justify what I have done to anyone else because, in the end, I have to live in this body. Since breast reconstruction after cancer surgery is covered by insurance, I could even justify it from a financial perspective. I needed to get out of my head and listen to my heart. When I finally did, I realized that choosing not to reconstruct out of fear of being judged for having implants is no more authentic than choosing reconstruction for fear of being flat-chested. Certainly, either path is honorable because navigating breast cancer is brave, period. Desiring breast reconstruction does not mean that I caved in to society's ideals of what a woman's body image should be; it does not mean I'm weak. I would actually have to make an argument for quite the opposite. Willingly choosing to endure several more surgeries, anesthesia, additional blood draws, IVs, sleepless nights and discomfort only meant that I was strong, and with each step, I only got stronger and more determined. I have learned much about myself during this process. I had always viewed myself as the sissy girl weakling, and I made a surprising discovery, that I'm actually tough as nails.

With my mind settled on rebuilding what cancer was taking from me, I was able to return my focus to what really counted in my life. I was able to welcome myself back home, perhaps a little modified, but healthy, and just as much a woman as before. I kept my thoughts positive because I have learned that negativity is a cancer of the soul that spreads like the flu, and I was finished with being sick.

During this journey, as I waited in different doctors' offices, I encountered many other women walking the same path as I. Each of them revealed incredible courage and strength, and touched places deep inside my feminine soul. I celebrate each and every one of these women; we are bosom buddies that will always be a connected sisterhood tied together by a pink ribbon.

# BEFORE YOUR SURGERY—
## Patient's suggestions

Nothing is worse than the feeling of being helpless and having to depend on other people to do things for you. While you are recovering, you are going to need assistance, but with good planning, you can be more independent when you get home from the hospital. This will make things not only easier on you, but also on other family members. When Mom is down, the entire household seems to fall apart. If you live alone, than the following will be especially important for you, although I highly recommend that you have someone stay with you, at least for the first few nights.

Usually, you will have a few days before your surgery to prepare while the doctors coordinate their schedules with the hospital, so make the most of them. You will have strict lifting and stretching restrictions, and it is important that you follow those directions. I'm listing here just a few small things that you can do to make your recovery time easier on you and your family members:

- If you have a dog or cat, you will be unable to lift a large bag of pet food or kitty litter. Take the time to prepackage these items into small bags that are no heavier than a pound.

- What is your regular beverage—soda, juice or milk? These containers will be too heavy for you to lift and then pour. You may even find it difficult to navigate the twist tops the first few days. Buy yourself cans of soda or juice boxes in individual serving sizes.

- Grab a six-pack of ginger ale, just in case you have any problems with nausea.

- Purchase food and plan as many easy meals as you can in advance. Cook and freeze them in single-serving containers, so that they can be heated up in the microwave.

- Do an extra thorough house cleaning because you will not be able to vacuum or do laundry. On some level, you should be able to relax and enjoy the break from regular household duties. It's nice to be waited on, but when the house gets messy or things aren't done the way you like them to be, it can get stressful. Just remember that you don't want to do something stupid and compromise your health and reconstruction; you aren't superwoman.

- Before you go to the hospital, put clean sheets on your bed; you'll appreciate them when you get home.

- Buy yourself a few good books or magazines; you'll actually have the time to relax and read them.

- If you knit or crochet, buy a few skeins of yard and dig out the knitting needles from storage now, so you have a project to do.

- Buy comfortable sleepwear, either nightgowns or pajamas; just make sure that they button down the front. You will have a hard time pulling garments over your head, especially if you are undergoing bilateral surgery. Keep in mind that the first week or so, you will also have drains that will need to be pinned onto your top.

- Purchase a few new shirts in advance; look for button-down or zippers. You will most likely go down a size in shirts, depending on your current breast size.

- Purchase a pair of open-back slippers and a pair of shoes that you can also just slip on without having to bend over.

- Purchase a soft cup-less bra, one that will offer you a little support but won't cut into you. This is the kind of bra that is made to sleep in. You don't want a tight sports bra.

- If you can set up the night table next to your bed with comfort items placed within arm's reach, you'll be happy when you arrive home from the hospital. Stock up the nightstand with tissues, lip balm, hand lotion, reading materials, crossword puzzle book and pen, phone and TV remote. When you get home, you can just crawl in and relax.

- If you don't have extras in the house now, purchase several more pillows for your bed. You will need one for under your legs and two more to tuck yourself in on your sides under your arms.

- Purchase a measuring cup, and place with it a piece of paper and pen, so you don't have to run around gathering up these items when you need them. You will be required to empty your drains three times a day and measure the volume; your doctor will need this information.

- Make arrangements with someone dependable, who can drive you to some of your follow-up appointments with the plastic surgeon. You will not be able to drive for a few weeks.

- Purchase dry shampoo; if you can't wash your hair, at least you can spray it to freshen it up, which will make you feel better.

- If you have young children, make arrangements for babysitting.

- Purchase comfort items, from favorite snacks to special toiletry items, anything that will make you feel just a little bit better. This is the time to spoil yourself; you deserve it.

- If it's financially possible, pay all your monthly bills, so you don't have to worry about doing that.

It is normal to feel anxious before any kind of surgery. Getting your house in order and enlisting friends and family to help you care for children and help with household chores can allow you to relax. The most important thing is that, after surgery, you get plenty of rest in order for your body to heal. Knowing everything is taken care of in advance will give you the peace of mind you need.

# MASTECTOMY SURGERY—
## What the doctor will tell you

You'll be moved to the recovery room after mastectomy surgery, where staff will monitor your heart rate, body temperature and blood pressure. If you are in pain or feel nauseous from the anesthesia, let someone know so that you can be given medication.

You'll then be admitted to a hospital room. Hospital stays for mastectomy average three days or fewer. If you have a mastectomy and reconstruction at the same time, you may be in the hospital a little longer.

Before you leave the hospital, your surgeon or nurse will give you information about recovering at home:

- Taking pain medication: Your surgeon will probably give you a prescription to take with you when you leave the hospital. You might want to get it filled on your way home or have a friend or family member get it filled for you as soon as you are home.

- Caring for the bandage (dressing) over your incision: Ask your surgeon or nurse how to take care of the mastectomy bandage. The surgeon may ask that you not try to remove the bandage, and instead wait until your first follow-up visit so that he or she can remove the bandage.

- Caring for a surgical drain: If you have a drain in your breast area or armpit, the drain might be removed before you leave the hospital. Sometimes, however, a drain stays inserted until the first follow-up visit with the doctor, usually one to two weeks after surgery. If you're going home with a drain inserted, you'll need to empty the fluid from the detachable drain bulb a few times a day. Make sure your surgeon gives you instructions on caring for the drain before you leave the hospital.

- Stitches and staples: Most surgeons use sutures (stitches) that dissolve over time, so there's no longer any need to have them removed. But occasionally, you'll see the end of the suture poking out of the incision like a whisker. If this happens, your surgeon can easily remove it. Surgical staples — another way of closing the incision — are removed during the first office visit after surgery.

- Recognizing signs of infection: Your surgeon should explain how to tell if you have an infection in your incision and when to call the office.

- Recognizing signs of lymphedema: You will be given information on taking care of your arm and being alert to signs of lymphedema.

- When you can start wearing a prosthesis or resume wearing a bra: The site of mastectomy surgery, and especially mastectomy with reconstruction, needs time to heal before you can wear a prosthesis or bra. Your doctor will tell you how long you may need to wait.

At-home recovery from mastectomy

It can take a few weeks to recover from mastectomy surgery, and longer if you have had reconstruction. It's important to take the time you need to heal.

In addition to your surgeon's instructions, here are some general guidelines to follow at home:

- Rest. When you get home from the hospital, you will probably be fatigued from the experience. Allow yourself to get extra rest in the first few weeks after surgery. You may experience fatigue from time to time in the early months after surgery.

- Take pain medication as needed. You will probably feel a mixture of numbness and pain around the breast incision and the chest wall, if you feel the need, take pain medication according to your doctor's instructions. Consult your doctor to learn more about managing chest pain, armpit discomfort and general pain.

- Take sponge baths until your doctor has removed your drains and/or sutures. You can take your first shower when your drains and any staples or sutures have been removed. A sponge bath can refresh you until showers or baths are approved by your doctor.

- Continue doing arm exercises each day. It's important to continue doing arm exercises on a regular basis to prevent stiffness and to keep your arm flexible.

- Have friends and family pitch in around the house. Recovery from mastectomy can take time. Ask friends and family to help with meals, laundry, shopping, and childcare. As your body heals, make sure you don't take on more than you can handle.

- You may have "phantom sensations" or "phantom pain" in the months after mastectomy. As nerves reconnect, you may feel a weird crawly sensation, you may itch, you may be very sensitive to touch, and you may feel pressure. Your discomfort may go away by itself, or it may persist, but you will adapt to it. Acetaminophen and ibuprofen usually can address the pain related to this type of nerve injury.

# DOWN TO THE BONE—
## Patient's view of the mastectomy

Obviously, before reconstruction can begin, we must first undergo the mastectomy. That morning, as I dressed for the hospital, I silently and briefly grappled with whether the path of least resistance would be to peel myself back to the bone, and bravely stay with a ballerina-type body forever, because it seemed I had so much ahead of me. I lingered in front of the mirror after my shower trying to grasp what would be my very last look at them. I tried to stay emotionless and move gracefully forward with the replication of what I was about to lose.

I had been secretly mourning the imminent loss of my breasts, but I would not have admitted that to anyone. During the car ride to the hospital, I began to think about them, and I realized that we had always had a love-hate relationship. I'd come to realize that, for me, saying goodbye to my breasts also meant letting go of what we had been through together, my past, but certainly not my womanhood. I've forgiven them for the embarrassment caused by their sudden and significant growth in my pre-teens, and for the shrinking they did when I lose weight in my 30's. I remembered the pain I had when they were grossly engorged with milk after giving birth to my daughter. At that time, they seemed to be nothing short of the size of watermelons. I remembered covering them with ice packs hoping the milk would disappear because I chose not to breastfeed, something I actually regretted. I reminisced about their abrupt deflation, which left them saggy and limp with the new added bonus of stretch marks. I thought of how my areolas had almost doubled in size due to my breasts breaking down and just falling, and how I had honestly needed a breast lift 20 years earlier. The reality was, they were no longer pretty. I could never justify spending the money on a breast lift. I always put other things first, even though I was growing extremely self-conscious about their aged appearance, especially when I had to wear a bathing suit in public. Still, with all the negatives, they were my breasts, and on some level, I still loved them. We had plenty of good times together too, growing into my own sexuality, transitioning from a child into a woman. I would often stuff them up into a pretty push-up bra to create nice full cleavage, and then wear a low-cut blouse. Perhaps I felt even a slight feeling of pride because they were home grown and more than ample in size. Only a female can completely understand the power those mounds of fat have over a man. For a woman, there is at least a small part of her identity that is connected to her mammary glands.

On the brink of a momentous change, by the time I reached the hospital for admission, I had finally made peace and let go of "the girls." I turned all my thoughts into positive ones. I empowered myself by starting to think in terms of what I would be gaining, not what I was losing. I told myself that the only thing I was losing was stupid cancer, and I certainly didn't want to keep that. Sure, I would be without breasts during the transition period, but when all of this was finished, I would be reclaiming that part of my body. I would have a new pair, a perky set, and I would feel and look like a million bucks. This was, in a way, almost turning back the hands of time. I would have breasts placed back where nature had intended them to be, and my insurance company would be paying for my boob job.

In essence, I think I discovered my courage that morning, which was probably the time that I would need it the most. When I signed in, and they called my name to go back to pre-op, I jumped up from my seat, walked swiftly with purpose, ready to move forward; I was strong and confident.

They did all the normal pre-op stuff to me: chest X-ray had my blood drawn, and an IV was placed into my hand. Then a young man wearing scrubs came to get me to take me down to what they called *nuclear*. This was something I hadn't been prepared for; it was a total surprise. The purpose of explaining all of this to you is not to frighten you. I want you to be prepared for it. I want you to know why they are going to do this to you and what it was like to go through. It wasn't horrible to go through physically; I just would have preferred to be mentally ready first, instead of having it thrown at me unexpectedly. I guess I just like to know what's coming. I knew that the surgeon would be removing at least one of my lymph nodes during the surgery, and I guess I had just assumed he would deal with it once he was inside. It was then explained to me that the reason I was being sent down the hall to nuclear was to prepare me for that part of the surgery, in order to help the surgeon find the lymph node or nodes that needed to be removed. The actual removal of the lymph node would take place during the mastectomy surgery, so that a sentinel node biopsy could be done. The obvious reason for removing a lymph node is to determine if cancer cells have metastasized (spread) beyond the original tumor or mass area, which also helps the doctors determine the actual stage of your breast cancer; 1, 2, 3, 4, or 5.

The radiologist quickly injected my areola with four needles. If you picture the areola as the face of a clock, the needles were put in at the positions of 12 o'clock, 3 o'clock, 6 o'clock and 9 o'clock. Each one felt like a small bee sting, which lasted for only a second or two. He injected me with a blue radioactive dye. I was given a hand massager to use on my breast for approximately 15 minutes, which would help the dye spread around in the breast. I had a slight burning sensation within the breast, which was completely tolerable. Then I was given a CT scan for the purpose of showing the surgeon the clump of lymph nodes receiving the dye. This indicates to him where your sentinel lymph node will be found, so that it can be removed. The surgeon will be looking for lymph nodes that have been stained with blue dye. Since lymph nodes can vary in size, some small as a pinhead, others large as a bean, the surgeon will be hunting through the skin and fat, looking for blue-dyed nodes with skill and judgment. Only one to three nodes are usually removed, unless many more are stained. These nodes are sent to the pathology lab to be examined for cancer.

Sometimes your surgeon will order a frozen section test for the nodes, in order to get results right then, while you are still on the operating table, which is what my surgeon did. If your nodes do contain cancer cells, you may have a full lymph node dissection immediately to find the full extent of lymph node involvement. If a frozen section is not ordered, and your nodes contain cancer, a full lymph node dissection will be done at a later time.

After the nuclear test had been completed, I was taken back to the pre-op holding area and saw my plastic surgeon. He had me stand up so that he could use a marker on my breasts to draw what appeared to be a complete roadmap of artwork on them. At that time, he explained that in order for me to receive the most optimal reconstruction results, the general surgeon who would be doing the actual double mastectomy needed to stay within all of his lines. I'm happy to say that he did. This is not always possible, depending on how and where your cancer has spread.

My mastectomy was performed by a general surgeon, and before I was closed up, the plastic surgeon placed skin expanders into my chest. This was the first step of my reconstruction. The combined surgery lasted approximately 6 ½ hours from start to finish. I had only one lymph node removed, which came back negative for cancer.

I naturally woke up feeling groggy, and I had compression sleeves on my legs to help with circulation, which didn't bother me. I had problems with extreme nausea the first evening in the hospital, and I received injections to keep me from getting sick to my stomach. This is a common occurrence, especially after a long surgery. Make sure you tell your nurses if you aren't feeling well; they will give you something to help. My pain level wasn't bad, and I remember thinking I had expected that it would be much worse.

Of course, one of the first things I did was attempt to have a look at my new chest. I had drains coming out of each of my armpit areas, with long tubing that had plastic bulbs at the end to create suction, which were filled with an orangey amber-colored liquid. I was completely bandaged with several layers of gauze and medical tape. Over that, I wore a tight white surgical Velcro vest that had been stuffed with endless wads of gauze where my breasts were only a few hours ago, and then the always-attractive standard hospital gown on top of that. I tugged at all of this in an attempt to have just a quick look, while my family members were scolding me to leave it alone. My daughter wasn't especially amused by my need to have just a look, and I could tell that she had no desire to see it. I secretly wondered if all of these layers were medically necessary or were just placed there to make it harder for me to take a peek at what I looked like underneath it all. Did the hospital staff fear that I would deem it all so hideous that I would leap from my bed and run down the hallway screaming in horror like a madman?

I was told that my first words upon waking were, "I'm ugly." Of course, this wasn't true, but a small part of me, only briefly, still felt like it was. My breasts were gone, and my chest looked like that of a little boy. I was told that no cancer had been found in my lymph nodes, my skin expanders were in, and I was already on the road to new boobs; and those thoughts made me smile. I knew those were the things I need to concentrate on.

I stayed in the hospital for four days before being discharged. Although, I had an IV in throughout my stay, I was offered a normal diet of solid food, but I didn't have much of an appetite for the first few days. I was able to get out of bed with some assistance and felt better once I put on some makeup and washed myself up. My family and friends all said that I looked well and, of course, I enjoyed their company, and support, plus the cards, books and flowers.

The first time I took a sponge bath in the small hospital bathroom, I capitalized on the opportunity to get a decent look at my chest. Surely the nurse had to know that, once I was unsupervised, I would do this. I was able to peel back most of the layers, with the exception of two thin long white taped bandages and a clear waterproof tape covering the exact incision areas. I was able to see the skin expanders in my chest, which looked like two donuts placed directly under the skin. Although my chest was sunken in, even with these foreign round objects, it really didn't look all that bad, in fact, nothing like the horror show I had conjured up in my mind. The top part of my body seemed so small, childlike in a way, and gave the impression that I had lost a lot of weight. It made me wonder what my natural double DDs had actually weighed because I felt thin. Upon discharge, I was sent home with instructions on how to care for my drains, prescriptions for pain and antibiotics to avoid infections. I also had an appointment to see my plastic surgeon in a few days.

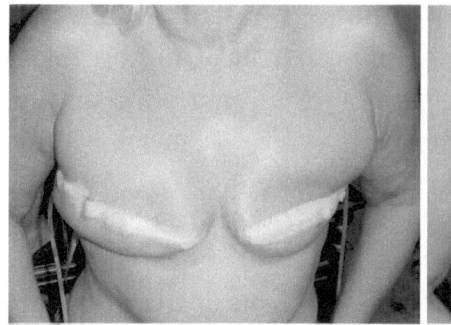 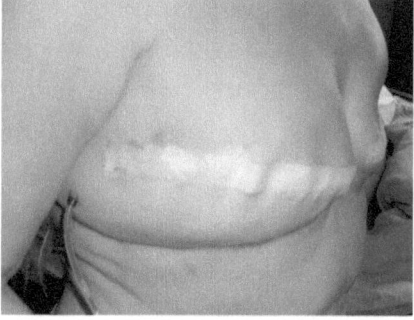

These were taken the day I came home from
the hospital after the mastectomy

# SKIN EXPANDERS—
## What the doctor will tell you

Early in the stages of the reconstruction process, you will most likely see your plastic surgeon weekly until the last drain has been removed. You cannot rush removing the drains; as bothersome as they may be, they are essential to proper wound healing. Generally, once an individual drain produces less than 20 to 30 cc's in a 24-hour period, your surgeon will remove it. In most patients, the drain removal does not hurt.

You will have tissue expanders in your chest for several weeks or even months. A tissue expander is a temporary device that is placed on the chest wall deep to the pectoral's major muscle. This may be done immediately following the mastectomy or as a delayed procedure. The purpose of the expander is to create a soft pocket to contain the permanent implant. Tissue expanders are available in a variety of shapes and sizes.

At the time of the initial post-mastectomy reconstruction operation, when it is first positioned on the chest wall, the tissue expander is partially filled with saline. Within a few weeks after this surgery, once the patient has healed, expansion can be started as an office procedure. The process of expansion takes place at one-, two—or three-week intervals over the course of several months. The amount of fluid that is placed into the expander at the time of the initial surgery will also determine how many expansions are required later. Today, with the use of a dermal matrix, the surgeon can usually place a higher volume of saline during the initial surgery. This may decrease the number of expansions needed later.

Most expanders have a fill port that is built into the front of the device. This port is accessed with a needle through the skin. Expansion takes about one minute, and the amount of fluid that can be injected is limited by the tightness of the patient's skin. A typical volume for each expansion procedure is 50 cc's of saline (about 10 teaspoons).

Most patients do not have significant discomfort or pain after expansion. Discomfort can generally be managed with acetaminophen, and the tightness should subside within 24 hours.

Once expansion is completed, then the patient will be medically cleared for the next operation, and the second stage of reconstruction is performed. It is important to remember that everyone is different, and we all heal at our own pace. What works for some may not work for others.

# FILL 'EM UP—Patient's view
## of the skin expanders

During your first few days home from the hospital, you should be resting or at least attempting to rest. I had an appointment with my plastic surgeon a few days after leaving the hospital, and I hoped he would remove my drains, but no such luck; I needed them in for another week. My hospital discharge papers stated that I wasn't allowed to take a shower until after I had my first visit with the doctor. It was a little scary to shave my armpits because they were completely numb. I wasn't sure if I had done a good job or even if I nicked myself with the razor. This is something that over time you get used to, having no feeling in that area, and learning how much pressure you need with the razor. To make it a little bit easier, you may want to start shaving in front of the mirror until you get the hang of it.

I washed up the best I could in the sink, but my hair was becoming a major problem, and I didn't want to go out looking and feeling like a grease ball. I seriously needed to do something about it, and quickly. I wasn't able to bend over the kitchen sink to wash it, and the can of dry shampoo wasn't working to my satisfaction, but I came up with the perfect solution. I had my daughter take me to the salon where I was able to sit in the chair and put my head back to have it washed. The hairdresser was slightly intimidated not only by the drain tubes, but by the sheer length of my hair. She actually told me that she had never worked on hair this long before. She suggested that I cut it, to make it easier during the next few months, foolish mortal. I made it clear to her that under no circumstances would I even consider such a thing, and that I just wanted her to wash and comb it out. I live in Florida and this was May, so it was hot enough outside that my hair would air-dry on the way to my doctor's appointment. She looked less than enthused; nevertheless, she did as I requested, and I tipped her well, which seemed to change her attitude. It took forever for her to comb all of the knots out of my hair, but I felt so much better when I left there with shiny, squeaky-clean hair. Now I could go to the doctor and at least feel human.

Several times a day, I had been squeezing the bulbs of the drains and measuring the output of liquid, and each day it decreased. The drains were not painful, but a little annoying; they were slightly irritating where they came out of my body, especially if I made the mistake of brushing up against that area and the tube moved. I was disappointed that the doctor didn't take them out on my first visit. He explained to me that I was still putting out a lot of volume, and it was very important that all of this excess fluid be drained, or it would cause me other problems down the road. The good news was that he removed the clear bandaging, which left me with only a thin white strip of tape that covered just my incisions. He also gave me the go-ahead to begin showering. When I took showers that week, I would tie a belt around my waist, so that I could pin the bulbs of the drains onto it; that way, my hands were free to wash my body and my own hair.

A week later, on my second visit to the doctor, he removed my drains. Now, as much as I wanted to get them out, I had a great fear about how it would feel. I made the foolish mistake of searching for this on the Internet and read a few horror stories. One woman claimed that it burned, and another even insisted that she had the sensation of snakes running wild and flipping throughout her chest when the drains were pulled out. Let me assure you that for me, the drain removal was a cinch. The doctor asked me to take a deep breath, and the next thing I knew, the drain was out, which took only a few seconds. I was shocked and greatly relieved, plus happy the drains were gone. I felt absolutely nothing at all, not inside or even at the area near my armpits where the drains had exited my body.

In the ensuing days, I was struggling to get much needed sleep, until I discovered the pillow trick. When you have chest expanders in, sleeping on your belly or your side is just not going to happen. The only way to sleep is on your back. If you are naturally a back sleeper you have it made, but if you aren't, this can cause a problem. Even though I knew I had no choice but to sleep on my back, falling asleep was a problem because I just wasn't comfortable. Once I managed to finally succumb from complete and utter exhaustion, my body did its normal natural thing, and I would attempt to turn on my side while I was out cold. This always ended the same way; I had a rude awakening. Expanders aren't fixed in a permanent spot, so they can and will shift. When one of them manages to land on top of the chest bone, it hurts. Luckily, you can do something about it. The minute this happens (and believe me, you will know when it happens), place two fingers directly on the area of pain, and massage it off the chest bone—ah, total relief. I had this happen to me once while I was in a store shopping. Instinctively my hand flew inside my halter top, straight to the area of pain, and I gave myself a five second massage and I don't know who was happier, me for relieving my pain, or the man down the aisle from me who witnessed me rubbing my own boob mound. Judging how his face changed from a jaw drop to a smile, I think it might have been him.

It took me a few weeks to figure out a way to stop myself from trying to turn in my sleep. I placed one pillow directly under the back of my knees. Then I took two other pillows and tucked them under my armpits and down my side lengthways. I would tuck these pillows into my side as tightly as possible and then place my arms on top of the pillows. This not only proved to be a comfortable position, but the pillows stopped me from turning during the night.

The following week, I returned to the plastic surgeon's office to have my first fill. This is a painless procedure and takes only a few minutes. A needle is placed through the skin into the expander, and saline solution fills it up. I had 50cc's each week for 10 weeks in a row, filling my expanders to their maximum capacity. My motto throughout was, "Go big or go home." I wanted the largest implant made for breast reconstruction: 800cc's, a full D cup, a size smaller than what my natural breasts had been. I admit that if a larger implant had been available, I would have been all in.

All doctors are different and all patients are different; you may have your fill-ups done every week or every other week. You may be injected with only 25cc's at a time or 50cc's or perhaps even more than that. All of this depends on your doctor, how well you tolerate the fills, what size implant you desire and how well your skin is stretching.

I would watch as my expanders were actually being injected. It was strange to visibly see them grow. I felt like an adolescent again, except this time, I was rapidly growing breasts right before my eyes, and I decided what their final size would be, not nature. With this comes some growing pains, or as the expression goes, no pain no gain. Although having your fills done is not in itself painful, because you don't even feel the needle going into the skin, you will feel extremely tight after each one. As the expanders grow, so will the mounds on your chest, but don't expect them to be perfectly shaped breasts. They were slightly irregular in shape; however, they were clearly doing their intended job, which is stretching skin, and creating pockets to hold the implants. As the expanders grew, they became even harder to the touch, nothing like the feel of a natural breast or implant. I overheard one woman in the doctor's office refer to them as "rocks in her chest." That kind of made me chuckle because her description as dead accurate.

I was a little concerned that the right one was larger than the left, but my doctor assured me that this wasn't a problem and, in fact, it was common. On my last fill, I had the normal 50cc's placed into the right one and then 100cc's put into the left one. That was a rough week, definitely the most uncomfortable one, but it was my last week of having injections into the expanders, and I sucked it up, knowing that my time with them was coming to an end. I preferred to be tighter for one week by doubling up, rather than having the expanders for an extra week. At this point, I really wanted them out.

What does it feel like to have skin expanders in your chest? Every year, I go to the renaissance fair and dress up as a wench. My costume has a tight corset, which always gave me awesome cleavage. After driving an hour to get there and wearing the corset all day while walking around, it's always a great relief to unlace it and take it off for the drive home. Skin expanders feel like you are wearing a corset inside your body, except you don't have the option of taking it off. I had days that I wished I could have just five minutes without this skin expander "corset", and on other days, I completely forget that I even had them inside of me. Sometimes it can be almost a claustrophobic type feeling, especially in the very beginning. This is where you need to be mentally tough, but you can do it. You must tell yourself that this is temporary, and as each day passes, you will be one day closer to getting them out. I kept a calendar on my desk during this time, and I would note each fill as I had it, counting the weeks and then days, which helped me, especially when I reached the halfway point. I would tell myself, if I keep these in just X amount of days, it will be the difference between living a lifetime as a B cup or a D cup. I looked back at my calendar, and counted out that I had skin expanders for 81 days. Some days passed by quickly and others did not, but it was worth the end result.

The first few hours after a fill were the worst ones, as far as the feeling of being tight. I discovered that when I kept myself super busy mentally, I would forget that I even had them in my chest. Do anything you can to keep your mind occupied. Sitting and watching TV isn't going to work; your brain needs more stimulation or your mind will only focus on how uncomfortable you are. My mother would take me for my fills, and we started going straight to the casino afterwards. I would sit at a slot machine for several hours, and my mind was being entertained, which helped me avoid dwelling on the tightness. Each day afterward I felt better and better, and then as my skin stretched, I became more comfortable again; at that point, unfortunately, it was usually time to get my next fill.

After the first one or two fills, I was afraid that my expanders would cause my incisions to literally rip open. I envisioned this happening and the expanders popping out. This was a silly fear and something that just doesn't happen.

I was concerned about the possibility that I would end up with terrible stretch marks from this procedure. Every night, I would rub a good moisturizing lotion into my expanders and the skin surrounding them, taking care not to put any lotion over or into the actual incisions. I can't really say for sure if this prevented me from getting stretch marks, but it probably didn't hurt either. I'm happy to say that I have absolutely none.

When I had the expanders in my chest, I held my upper body stiff. I would routinely encounter other woman going through the same process at the plastic surgeon's office, and I could tell, just from looking at them, what stage they were in of their reconstruction. It's a distinct look, the way we all seemed to hold an awkward rigid position, almost as if we were wearing some kind of invisible upper body brace.

The expanders also make driving a bit of a challenge. I was fine when going straight, but making turns was a little bit harder than I thought it would be. Don't rush to get behind the wheel; let a few weeks go by before you even attempt it. After you've driven a few times, you'll get the hang of how you need to navigate the steering. If you aren't comfortable driving or feel that your reaction time would be too slow, then use common sense and get someone to chauffeur you around.

Now on the bright side, yes, there always has to be a bright side of things, I was able to capitalize on having small firm breasts during the expander period. The one thing that flat-chested woman can do that large-breasted woman can't do is to go braless. This is something I hadn't experienced since the age of 11. I dug deep into my closet and pulled out every single halter top, spaghetti strap shirt and strapless top that I owned. During the expander period, I wore every item of clothing that had previously required the addition of an uncomfortable tight strapless bra. Since I had no nipples, I didn't have to worry about headlights showing through either. It was an amazing time of freedom, having no straps digging into my shoulders, and I took full advantage of it.

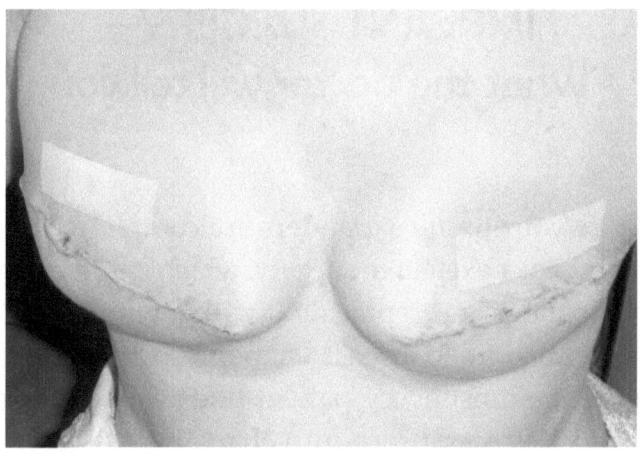

This was taken after three fill injections, seven more to go

# IMPLANT SURGERY—
## What the doctor will tell you

Once your tissue expanders are completely filled, you are ready for your exchange surgery, which involves removing the skin expander and replacing it with an implant. This will create a more refined breast shape. You can rest assured knowing that almost every patient finds expander exchange to be a much easier procedure than the mastectomy and expander placement. The tight feeling caused by the tissue expander disappears and is replaced by the softer feel of the final implant. Although you may still awaken from surgery with feelings of tightness across your chest, this pain will ease quickly, and you will likely not have any drains.

Keep in mind that it takes time for swelling to go down and for your body to heal after surgery. If you are having a procedure done to your opposite breast, such as a reduction or a lift, you will require more time to heal. Almost always, these surgeries are done as outpatient procedures, requiring only about an hour and a half for each breast. Then you will stay for a short while in recovery and be sent home. If your surgeon has asked you to keep a surgical or sports bra on following surgery, trying to sneak a peek isn't worth it. No one can wrap or bandage you better than your surgeon or the nurse, and it may be preferable to do the unveiling in your surgeon's office. It is important that you keep your bandages clean and dry, so no showering is allowed until after you have seen the doctor.

As part of your reconstruction recovery, it is essential that you adhere to all lifting restrictions provided by your surgeon. You should not engage in any strenuous activity. Doing laundry, vacuuming the house and lifting heavy objects may result in wound healing problems.

Taking medications: Your surgeon will probably give you some prescriptions, one for pain management and another which will be an antibiotic that lowers the risk of infection. You should have them filled on your way home or have a friend or family member get them for you as soon as you are home.

Every surgery involves risks; women who choose to have breast reconstruction using implants face the possibility of complications.

Risks:

- Capsular contracture—This is a condition in which the scar surrounding the implant tightens. The implant or scar tissue may need to be removed if this occurs.

- Rupture or deflation of the implant—Saline implants can rupture suddenly while the silicone implants can deflate over a long period of time. This is very rare with the newer implants.

- Delayed wound healing.

- Poor reaction to anesthesia — Possible reactions include, nausea, vomiting, dizziness, blurred vision, headache, itching, urinary difficulties, and chest infection.

- Infection

- Bleeding

# EXCHANGE ME—Patient's view
## of the implant surgery

This was the day I had been really looking forward to, getting those skin expanders out and having my implants put in. I had it noted in bold black magic marker on my calendar because it seemed much more important than any birthday or holiday, at least to me it did. The day that I had strived for was here, I had finally reached my goal date, and the days of the countdown were over. The worst of it was behind me now, and the rest of the reconstruction would be easy sailing.

I arrived early at the surgical center, had the normal blood draw and an IV placed in my hand, and off to surgery I went, but this time I was very excited. I'm not sure what I was happier about, having the expanders removed or getting the implants; either way, it was a win.

The surgery didn't take very long, about three hours. I woke up in recovery and stayed for only about two hours before they sent me home. Once again, I quickly discovered that I had been heavily bandaged and wearing a white Velcro surgical vest stuffed with gauze, which didn't allow me a preview of my new investments.

I didn't feel any pain at all with this surgery or during its recovery. In fact, what I recall the most was the feeling of my upper body relaxing and actually being comfortable. The implants felt like a cushion between my skin and chest bone, such a big difference.

The first night I thought, "Finally I can get rid of all of these pillows, and sleep on my side," but that didn't happen. I was a little sore from the surgery and slightly swollen, probably more than I had actually realized. I ended up tucking myself back in again, with my usual extra pillows, realizing that I still needed to sleep on my back, which I did for two more weeks.

I was aware of the implants in my chest, more than I thought I would be. I had thought they would be like my old boobs, that I would feel like my old self again, and be completely comfortable. The initial discomfort concerned me a little. It took about two weeks for the implants to become part of me, as swelling went down. At this point, I lost the feeling of having something foreign in my body and they truly felt like a part of me.

I had been sent home with instructions not to get my bandages wet. I was back to, once again, taking sponge baths and having greasy dirty hair. Sometimes it feels like two steps forward and one step back. The morning of my doctor's visit, I decided to try something new. I had told myself that if this didn't work, it probably wouldn't be a problem anyway, because the doctor would be removing the bandages that day. I was desperate to wash my hair, and I thought hard about how I could accomplish that without having to go back to the salon. I wanted and needed a real shower. Every woman knows the feeling I'm talking about, and how alive you feel after you've showered and washed your hair; it just makes you feel human again. I removed the Velcro vest and mounds of gauze that it had been stuffed with. This left me with two white bandages, covering the incisions. I tied a large black garbage bag across my chest tightly, as if it were a tube top. Then I took another precaution; I used 2-inch-thick masking tape straight across the top of the black bag, placing half of the tape on the baggie and the other half directly on my skin to create a waterproof seal. I took a shower, washed my hair and felt great. When I removed my tape and garbage bag, my bandages were dry, so my idea worked like a charm, and I was sorry that I hadn't thought of it sooner. I would use this shower trick again, after my areola and nipple surgeries.

Before I got dressed, I stood looking at myself in the mirror; this was the first really good look that I had gotten. I couldn't help but notice how high my new breasts were and that they were perfectly shaped. I actually thought to myself, gee, I never realized this is where breasts actually should be. I hadn't really seen the very top of my ribcage in years because my old saggy breasts slung down and lay over that part of my body. I felt them; they weren't hard, they were soft, and seemed very similar to normal breast tissue, which really shocked me. Plus they looked wonderful, although I admit, it was just a little odd to see them with no nipples or areolas.

I decided on the silicone breast implants, which I'm very happy with. I feel that they are superior to saline implants.

I went to the doctor, and he removed the bandages and a few tiny stitches. I would return a week later for a checkup, and to find out the date of my next surgery, which would be about six weeks later. My breast reconstruction was moving right along, and with the implants in, I looked completely normal in all of my clothing.

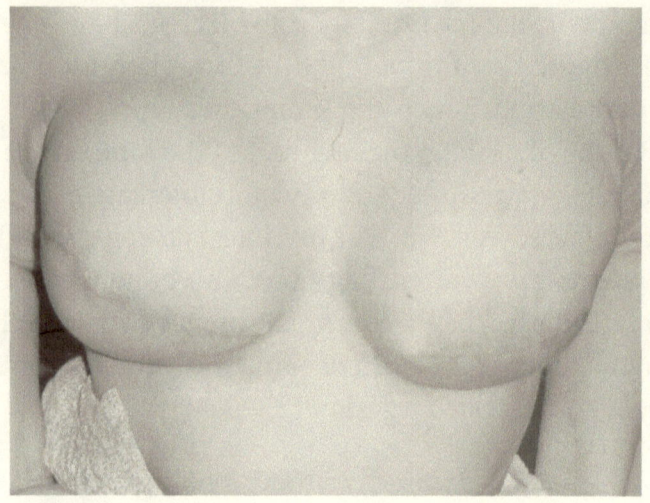

This was taken a week after my expander/.
implant exchange surgery

# NIPPLE & AREOLA RECONSTRUCTION—
## What the doctor will tell you

After you have had your implant surgery, and are happy with the size and shape of your reconstruction, and time has passed for you to heal, you may want to consider having nipple and areola reconstruction.

The nipple and areola created by your surgeon will not be like your natural nipple. It will not react to temperature or touch by flattening or becoming larger, and it will most likely not have any feeling. This is often the last phase of breast reconstruction, and it makes the breast look more natural and aesthetically pleasing. Depending on the type of breast reconstruction, reconstructed nipples may appear more or less perky than others. Some women are content to go without a nipple and areola on their reconstructed breast.

Nipple and areola reconstruction can be accomplished with a variety of techniques. It depends on your surgeon and, to some degree, on whether an already existing nipple is being matched or if two matching nipples need to be reconstructed. The technique that involves the least alteration of the overall shape of the breast mound is the skate flap. The skate flap technique involves cutting some of the skin and soft tissue on the newly reconstructed breast and folding the tissue like a Japanese origami puzzle to create the nipple. Most of these procedures involve taking skin from a local flap of the reconstructed breast and using a skin graft from another location of the body, usually your inner thigh or abdomen, to create the areola.

The surgeon will use a marker to draw on your breast, and perhaps the donor site on another area of your body, to show where the incisions will be made. You will be asked to stand up while this happens to assist in proper placement of your areola and nipple.

In some cases, the surgeon may also decide to enhance the nipple projection by adding fat grafts or even a core of dermal matrix product, a skin substitute such as AlloDerm, into the reconstructed nipple so that it doesn't flatten out.

This is an outpatient procedure, and surgery will usually last about 2 hours for each breast.

Areola tattooing will be offered later on after you heal. It is performed in an office setting, and usually painless. There are a variety of flesh-tone colors available to create a natural-looking areola. Keep in mind that most tattoos will fade as much as 40% over time and may need to be reapplied after a few years.

The success of nipple reconstruction surgery depends largely on aftercare. The patient must follow the surgeon's post-operative instructions to ensure proper healing.

The doctor will give you pain medication and antibiotics as needed. You will not be able to get your dressings and stitches wet, so you should not shower.

Your reconstructed nipple will probably look pointed and somewhat larger in the beginning. After the stitches are removed or dissolve, the nipple will begin to flatten out and shrink in size.

# THE FULL EFFECT—Patients view of Nipple & Areola reconstruction

I was surprised to learn that both of my breasts would not be done together; it would end up being two separate surgeries. I had areola and nipple reconstruction done on my left breast first, and then six weeks later, I had surgery on the right one.

These were done in the hospital as an outpatient. I had all the normal routine pre-op work done, chest X-ray, blood draw and IV. Each surgery lasted approximately two and a half hours. I stayed in recovery for about an hour and then was sent home.

The nipple/areola area was heavily bandaged, so I couldn't get even a peek. Once again, I came home wearing one of those super attractive white surgical vests, which had been heavily stuffed with gauze for extra protection. As with my previous surgeries, I was naturally curious to see what I looked like, but because of the heavy surgical taping, I would be forced to wait until I saw the doctor about a week later.

I was given two prescriptions, one for pain and the other was an antibiotic. I was instructed not to shower or to get the bandages wet. Once again, I was able to defy this rule by using my black garbage bag shower trick. I actually admitted to my doctor after my last surgery that I had been doing this all along, because I just needed to be clean and wash my hair. He wasn't upset at all; in fact, he told me that it was a great idea, as long as my bandages stayed dry.

I was told that I needed to be extra careful about having someone or something bang into the nipple area during this time. While I was healing from these surgeries, I took extra care when I went any place crowded by either placing my purse on that side, to keep just a little distance, or I would have someone walk on that side of me, almost like a wall of protection.

Most likely because I always had this on my mind, I had a dream one evening during the healing process. In the dream, I saw myself peacefully sleeping and then waking up. As I pulled the covers back, I could see my new nipple and areola lying next to me on the bed, as if it had just fallen off. Then my little 4-pound male Yorkshire terrier dog, who had been sleeping at the foot of my bed, popped his head up and carefully looked back and forth at the nipple on the bed and then at my chest. From his facial expression and the way he cocked his head to one side, it was clear he too was entirely confused and dumbfounded. Finally, my dog actually spoke to me (it was a dream, OK?), and said, "Ah, I think that might be a problem." What struck me the most about this was, his voice was nothing I would have expected to come out of him, a deep males voice. I guess since he wears a hair bow, a blue one, I had expected it would have been a little higher in pitch. Now, for the record, although this clearly was a fear that I had deep down in my own subconscious, which is why I had this crazy dream, please understand that this can't really happen; the nipple and areola simply can't just fall off.

A week later, I was back in the plastic surgeon's office ready for the unveiling of my nipple and areola. The areola looked very good, but the nipple was swollen, gooey and bloody looking. My doctor cleaned up the area, and instructed me to apply Neosporin to the nipple and areola three times a day, and to keep it covered with a gauze pad. The nipple was slightly larger than I had expected. For some reason, I feared having nipples that were too big, which would give me permanent headlights. Just as my doctor had predicted, my nipple shrank in size over the next few weeks, to the ideal size.

My second nipple and areola surgery went exactly the same way. After seeing my doctor a few more times, he said I had graduated. He recommended that I follow up in about a year to have my areola tattooed, which I'm planning to do. I have come this far; I must see this to completion.

Having surgery can be scary, and after having a mastectomy and then implant surgery, maybe you have had enough. If you have decided to pass on the nipple and areola reconstruction, that is your choice to make; certainly no one will be able to tell from looking at you in clothing.

# TISSUE FLAP RECONSTRUCTION

There are several methods of breast reconstruction. Tissue flap surgery is another way for a plastic surgeon to rebuild the shape of your breast using your own skin, fat and muscle, which will be taken from another part of your body. These technical details of these procedures, at first glance, may seem overwhelming, but they shouldn't be if explained correctly. Basically, the differences between the different flap procedures have to do with where the donor tissue is being taken from, and how that tissue is actually removed by the surgeon.

Tissue flap Breast reconstruction usually requires more than one surgery. The first surgery is to create the breast and the second to create the nipple and areola. After you meet with your plastic surgeon, hopefully before your mastectomy, he can discuss which procedure is best for you.

Below are the different types of tissue flap reconstructions, which are named for the donor area of the body.

## TRAM (transverse rectus abdominis muscle)

The TRAM flap is probably the most common of the flap surgeries. The surgeon will take muscle and tissue from your lower belly and relocate it to the chest area to create a breast shape. The obvious benefit to this procedure is that it reduces the amount of fat and skin in the lower belly, which results in somewhat of a tummy tuck. The TRAM flap can decrease the strength in your belly, however, and may not be possible in women who have had abdominal tissue removed in previous surgeries. The TRAM Flap prodecure can be done using what's known as a pedicle flap, which simply means that the tissue is moved to the chest without cutting its original blood supply. The tissue is actually pulled under the skin up to the chest area and then attached. The other way of doing it would be using a free flap. In this technique the tissue is removed and the blood vessels are actually cut. After the flap is in place, the surgeon sews the blood vessels in the flap to blood vessels in the chest area. This requires careful surgery using a microscope (microsurgery) to reconnect tiny vessels.

## Latissimus dorsi (LD) flap

This is another type of pedicle flap surgery, in which the tissue is moved to the chest without cutting its original blood supply. Instead of taking tissue from the tummy, the surgeon uses muscle, fat and skin from the upper back. Some women may have weakness in their back, shoulder or arm after this surgery. The incision on the back is usually made at the bra line in order to make the resulting scar less visible. Sometimes, it is still necessary to use an implant to make the breast larger.

## Gluteal free flap

This is a free-flap procedure, which means the original tissue is removed from the donor area and the blood supply is cut. Muscle, fat and skin are removed from the buttocks to create a new breast. This is usually the best choice for thin women who don't have enough belly tissue for the other procedures.

## DIEP (deep inferior epigastric artery perforator) flap

This is a free flap procedure, which means the original tissue is removed from the donor area and the blood supply are cut. This is similar to the TRAM flap procedure because the surgeon will be taking fat and skin from the lower belly area, but this technique doesn't use any of the muscle. The benefit of this is that by saving muscle, the patient is less likely to experience belly weakness. Just like the TRAM flap procedure, this actually results in a tummy tuck. This procedure takes longer than the TRAM pedicle flap, which I discussed above, but causes less muscle weakness and causes fewer hernias.

## TUG flap (transverse upper gracilis or inner thigh)

This is a newer option for those who can't or don't want to use TRAM or DIEP flaps. This surgery uses the muscle and fatty tissue from along the bottom fold of the buttock that extends to the inner thigh. The skin, muscle, and blood vessels are cut and moved to the chest, using a microscope to connect the tiny blood vessels to their new blood supply. Obviously, women with thin thighs don't have much tissue here, so the very best candidates for this type of surgery are women whose inner thighs touch and who need a smaller or medium-sized breast. Sometimes there are healing problems due to the location of the donor site, but they tend to be minor and are easily treated. This option is not available everywhere.

All of these operations leave two surgical sites and scars, one where the tissue was taken from and one on the reconstructed breast. The scars will naturally fade over time, but they will never go away completely. In general, the tissue used in flap procedures behaves just like the rest of your body tissue. Because it is your own tissue, the new breasts may enlarge or shrink as you gain or lose weight. The advantage to having a flap is that you don't have to worry about replacing implants or rupturing implants. Breasts reconstructed using this method look and feel like natural tissue because they are natural tissue.

So if flap procedures are so wonderful, then why aren't all breast reconstruction surgeries done using this method? There are several reasons, but one major issue is that these procedures are all highly complex. All of these flap surgeries require a high level of skill to perform correctly, and most surgeons' training and experience leans much more heavily toward implant procedures. With flap surgery, the biggest challenges are to shape the breast in ways that balance well with the patient's body, and to create a reliable blood supply to keep the reconstructed breast tissues healthy. If you want a flap procedure, make sure that you have a surgeon with significant experience and knowledge in this area, preferably one that has done thousands of these procedures. Otherwise, you risk flap failure. Flap procedures aren't the kind of surgeries that an average plastic surgeon can successfully perform.

What is better: implants or flaps? Both are good; it just depends on which is best for your body. For the best breast reconstruction results, you must take into account your body type, fat distribution, details of your breast cancer, cancer treatments, past medical history, recovery time and personal aesthetic goals. Both implants and flaps have specific risks and benefits, and not every woman is a candidate for each procedure. This is a decision that must be made with your doctor. It is also important to note that your insurance may also have a say in which procedure you will have.

Occasionally, a combination of flap and implant is performed to achieve a woman's specific size goal. Generally in this case, the flap is performed first and an implant is then placed beneath the flap about six months later to augment the reconstruction.

## Having the flap surgery

The flap surgery is done as an inpatient procedure under general anesthesia. All flap procedures take several hours to complete. The doctor may only do one breast at a time; so a second surgery could be needed if you have had a double mastectomy. It is important to know that this surgery may require a blood transfusion.

You will wake up from your surgery feeling drowsy and will have bandages over the incisions, and also be wearing a tight surgical bra over that. You can expect to have drainage tubes in to collect fluid and prevent it from building up around the surgery sites. On average, you will have a five day hospital stay so that the doctor can be sure there is a good blood supply to the skin over the reconstruction.

You will experience soreness, redness and swelling in the breast as well as the areas where the donor tissue was taken from. Don't be alarmed; this is normal and understand that this swelling can last for several weeks. You will be given pain medicine and placed on an antibiotic to help prevent infection. As with implant breast reconstruction surgery, you will need to avoid strenuous activity or heavy lifting for at least six weeks or more. Remember that this is major surgery and needs to be treated as such. Take it easy during the recovery time; make sure that you understand the doctor's instructions and restrictions regarding your activities. Expect to be tired and sore for weeks to come as you recover. You will have stitches, most likely the absorbable suture type; that don't need to be removed.

Breast implant surgery is easier and quicker to recover from than tissue flap surgery. Most women who have tissue flap surgery are very happy with the final results, but you need to know that these surgeries are much longer and so is your recovery time. Some feel that flaps often result in a more natural-looking breast if done correctly, but that is just a matter of opinion. Others will argue that implants look better. Just like the implant surgery, flap breast reconstruction cannot restore the normal feeling to your breast, but with time, some feeling may return.

You are not considered a good candidate for flap procedures if you smoke, are in poor health or have any of the following problems: connective tissue disease, vascular disease, obesity, high blood pressure, or diabetes. These conditions put you are a higher risk for complications. Every surgery has risks, including the potential for infection, poor wound healing, bleeding or a bad reaction to the anesthesia. The added complications from flap breast reconstruction surgery are:

- Tissue death, called necrosis (if blood supply to the flap is not restored, which will result in the need for additional surgery)

- Abnormal scarring

- Muscle weakness from donor sites

- Collection of blood or clear fluid in the wound

- Prolonged time in surgery under anesthesia

- Ongoing pain or discomfort in the breast area

- Extended recovery and healing time

- Loss of sensation at the tissue donor site

- Abdominal wall hernia, muscle damage or weakness

- Difference in the size and shape of the breasts.

You will have to wait until you are healed before the second step of this process, nipple and areola reconstruction, can be completed.

# SKIN, NIPPLE AND AREOLA
# SPARING MASTECTOMY

In the cases of prophylactic (preventive) mastectomy or very low-grade breast cancers, a few doctors will give you the option of having skin, nipple and areola sparing mastectomies. The obvious advantage to this is that you may be able to eliminate the need to reconstruct the nipple and areola, plus, there is no need to have skin expanders. Preserving the nipple and areola can make the reconstructed breast appear more natural.

The decision to retain the nipple, areola and any additional skin is based upon a few important criteria's. Women with large tumors are not candidates for this surgery, because the cancerous area needs to be a minimum of 2 centimeters away from the tissue to be saved. Women with very large breasts tend to be poor candidates also because nipple displacement seems to be a problem with this kind of surgery. Woman who do not need a significant breast lift will have the best cosmetic results.

The incision to remove the breast tissue is commonly made around the areola, preserving it. The nipple and areola remain attached to the adjacent breast skin and an implant is then inserted. In layman's terms, I like to refer to this surgery as a scoop-out, because basically they are just removing breast tissue inside and leaving the outside of the breast as intact as possible.

Cancer cell biopsy (frozen section) is immediately taken from the tissue directly behind the nipple and areola. If this biopsy is negative, then the area can be preserved, but if it's positive, the nipple and areola need to be removed, and reconstruction of the nipple and areola will follow at a later time.

If you decide on this kind of mastectomy, you must understand that even though the nipple and areola are being saved, the area usually loses normal sensation due to resection of the nerves. Its shape can also change and perhaps even flatten as a result of the surgery. It is very unlikely the feeling will be as Mother Nature intended, so you must be realistic about your expectations.

A skin, nipple and areola sparing mastectomy can be combined with immediate breast reconstruction, and it usually is completed in about five or six hours, requiring a hospital stay of about three days. To save the nipple area, breast reconstruction must be performed immediately following the mastectomy.

As with any surgery, there are risks. Nipple sensation is usually significantly reduced, and sometimes the feeling is lost completely. The underside of the nipple and areola is shaved down to remove as much of the breast tissue as possible. This can sometimes compromise the blood supply to the tissue, which can cause healing problems. If the blood supply is just too damaged by the mastectomy, part or all of the nipple and areola can actually die. If this happens, it is removed to prevent wound healing complications, and a new nipple and areola are reconstructed at a later time.

This surgery is best for a woman who hasn't actually been diagnosed with breast cancer and is having a preventive mastectomy. Some doctors will not offer this surgery at all as an option. There is an added risk of cancer recurrence because you are keeping the skin, nipple and areola, which are all part of the breast. On the hand, many doctors will argue that it is a safe new procedure and that women who have it seem to do better mentally and emotionally. Only time will tell whether or not this is wise, because this hasn't been an option until fairly recently.

I'm certainly not a doctor, but for whatever it is worth, let me throw my own opinion in here. For the little you think you are gaining, or maybe the proper words should be *not losing*, it's not really worth the risk. You are having a mastectomy to get rid of breast tissue and cancer; get rid of the entire risk, not just most of it. I can tell you that nipple and areola reconstruction has really come a long way, and I think you would be very surprised at how good they really look. As I have said many times in the course of this book, in the end, you are the one who needs to make the final decision. Ask yourself the tough questions and then decide. I think I would be willing to go this route only if I were having a preventive mastectomy.

# INTERVIEW WITH DR. JOHN ROACH—
## Plastic surgeon

Dr. John Roach founded the Bayside Center for Plastic and Reconstructive Surgery in 2008. He received his Bachelor of Science Biology from State University of New York at Oneonta. He then went on to earn his Masters in Biomedical Science from Barry University, and later his Doctorate in Osteopathic Medicine from NOVA Southeastern University.

He earned his vast experience in general, plastic and reconstructive surgery by receiving training in numerous hospitals in Philadelphia and working with dozens of renowned surgeons. Dr. Roach's experience and knowledge led him to be named chief resident in plastic and reconstructive surgery at the Philadelphia College of Osteopathic Medicine.

Throughout his education and career, he has earned numerous honors. He was on the chancellor's list at the NOVA College of Osteopathic Medicine, and he was a member of the Sigma Sigma Phi National Honorary Osteopathic Fraternity. Dr. Roach received the H. Jeffrey Tourigian D. O. Memorial Scholarship Award, and he graduated from medical school with honors.

Dr. Roach is currently on the medical staff at Regional Medical Center Bayonet Point in Hudson, FL, and Medical Center of Trinity located in Trinity, FL.

Dr. Roach encourages realistic expectations through education, so that all patients know exactly what to expect from their procedure and their recovery process.

In his own words: "Studies show that breast cancer patients who undergo breast reconstruction have better outcomes, and we want women to understand all of their choices. There is an important decision to make between a mastectomy and a lumpectomy, and these choices can make a big difference during a breast reconstruction. There are choices, and we are dedicated to walking each of our patients through the entire process from start to finish."

O'Grady: What percentage of your practice is dedicated to breast reconstruction?

Dr. Roach: At least 50% of my practice is dedicated to strictly breast reconstruction, and it will always be that way.

O'Grady: Some doctors are doing nipple and skin sparing mastectomies. How do you feel about that?

Dr. Roach: This is something that is fairly new. It should only be done when a woman has a very small cancer, which is more than 2 centimeters away from the nipple. More research needs to be done long term. It is better suited for a woman who is having a prophylactic (preventive) mastectomy. It does pose challenges though, especially with larger breasts, as far as achieving the correct nipple and areola placement.

O'Grady: Will you do breast reconstruction on a woman who has received radiation treatments?

Dr. Roach: Yes, but it has to be done a little bit differently with skin grafting. One alternative is to utilize a tissue transfer such as a latissimus dorsi myocutaneous flap (LDMF)for implant reconstruction. The other alternative is to proceed with an autogenous flap, such as a TRAM flap.

O'Grady: How long do these implants last and will weight loss or weight gain have any effect on them?

Dr. Roach: It is recommended that implants should be exchanged every 10 years. With implant reconstruction, you can lose or gain weight and your breast size will not change.

O'Grady: What about with one of the flap procedures?

Dr. Roach: That is your own tissue; therefore, the breasts can change in size if you gain or lose weight.

O'Grady: We all know that smoking has detrimental health effects, but does it cause any other additional problems during breast reconstruction?

Dr. Roach: Yes, it's very bad; don't do it. Smoking during reconstruction increases complications such as infection or tissue death.

O'Grady: I know that you do breast reconstructions using implants and tissue flap procedures. Do you feel that one procedure is better than the other?

Dr. Roach: Flap reconstruction has more of an extensive recovery time than implant reconstruction, plus healing must take place in two areas of the body instead of just one.

Also, the technical complexity of the surgery has a prolonged surgical operation time. The preferred method is implant reconstruction, which I think has better cosmetic results.

O'Grady: Breast cancer doesn't discriminate; men get it too. Have you ever done breast reconstruction on a man?

Dr. Roach: That's a good question. No, I haven't done any reconstructions on men.

O'Grady: That really surprises me.

Dr. Roach: Well, you need to understand that the law under the Women's Health and Cancer Rights Act (WHCRA) only protects women; therefore, insurance companies don't have to pay for a man's reconstruction. Reconstruction on a man is actually considered to be cosmetic surgery.

O'Grady: Scars naturally fade over time, but is there anything a woman can do to help make her scars from these surgeries fade faster?

Dr. Roach: Sometimes, using Vitamin E oil can help to decrease the appearance of scars, but they will fade on their own in time.

O'Grady: After having breast reconstruction, do I still need to have a yearly mammogram?

Dr. Roach: That really is up to the woman's oncologist to make that decision. It's impossible for any surgeon to remove 100% of the breast tissue during a mastectomy; of course, we try to get all of it, but somewhere around 2 percent will still remain.

O'Grady: Does breast reconstruction make any recurring cancer harder to detect?

Dr. Roach: No, it makes no difference. Reconstructive surgery has not been shown to make it harder to detect cancer recurrence. There are several methods used to screen for cancer including an MRI.

If you would like to make an appointment with Dr. Roach, see contact information below:

Dr. John B. Roach Jr, DO
Bayside Plastic Surgery
Ballantrae Professional Center
17723 Hunting Bow Circle
Suite 101
Lutz, FL 33558
(727) 233-7307
**www.baysideplastics.com**

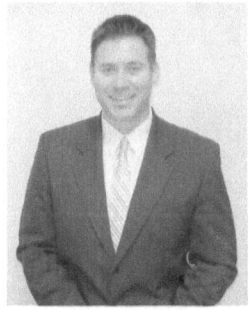

Dr. John Roach, Jr. DO

My personal experience with Dr. Roach and his staff was a positive one, from my consultation to "graduation." Below, you will find before and after pictures from my bilateral breast reconstruction, which was recently completed by Dr. John Roach. I believe my results were amazing, and the care I received from this doctor was more than any patient could ever ask for. I feel fortunate to have had him as my doctor, and I highly recommend him. He always maintained his professionalism even when faced with my own twisted sense of humor. I'm quite sure that I'm the only patient he had that asked if I should tweak my nipple to keep its projection; for the record, he didn't recommend it. I would also like to thank him for taking the time to do this interview; it's just another example of how available he is to his patients.

I did briefly struggle with the decision to put pictures of my own breasts in this book, but after careful consideration, I decided that since I've already bared my soul in so many ways, I see no reason why I shouldn't expose my breasts too.

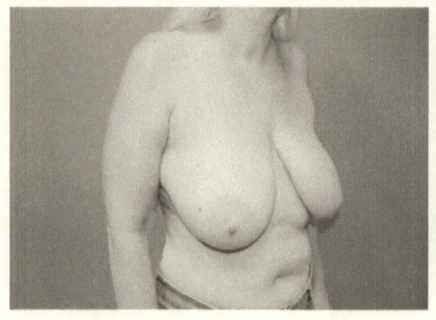
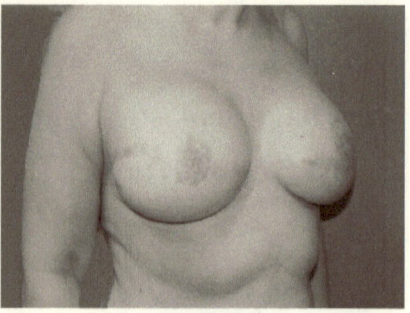

BEFORE                                        AFTER

Whatever you want to call them—breasts, boobs, boobies, bust, cans, tatas, hooters, tits, titties, the girls, the twins, honkers, second base, headlights, headlamps, high beams, knockers, jugs, puppies, funbags, airbags, gazongas, balloons, mammaries, melons, rack, bazookas, bazoomas, bosoms, boulders, cantaloupes, cha-chas, chumbawumbas, coconuts, grillwork, hood ornaments, milkshakes, mounds, muffins, moneymakers, pillows or torpedoes—it's so good to have them back.

# TATTOOING

After your nipple and areola surgery is completed, you will have to wait to have the areola tattooed pink. My doctor recommends waiting a year. If you decided against having nipple and areola reconstruction surgery, you can have a nipple and areola tattoo done. Of course, this will not give you any projection, but it will give you a nice appearance.

If you are a little bit daring, you have another option: getting an artisan tattoo. These work very well to cover a scar, which can partially mitigate a painful experience both emotionally and psychologically. Over time, your mastectomy and reconstruction scars will fade, but if you are self-conscious about them, there is a way to conceal them with fantastic skin art.

Tattoos are personal; almost all are custom designed, which means they come in a variety of styles, colors and sizes. Some breast cancer patients feel that getting a tattoo celebrates their inner strength and survival.

Prior to getting a tattoo, it is important to discuss the overall process and design options with a licensed and professional tattoo artist. Good design, planning and positioning, which takes into account the scar shape, size and type will result in a beautiful cover-up. Also, make sure that you discuss this with your doctor because he can advise you on when it is safe for you to take this step.

Look for a design that gives depth and doesn't rely solely on symmetry or an exact shape. Ask the artist to use a diversity of colors that can detract attention from the scar itself by allowing the eye to focus on the surrounding image.

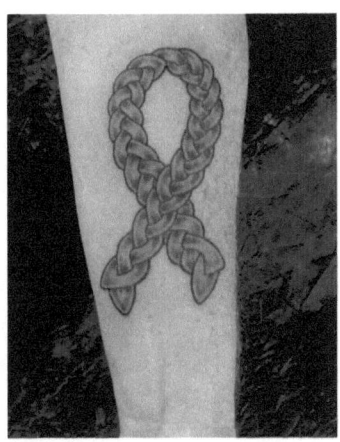

# INTERVIEW WITH PAT FISH—Tattoo artist

I had the pleasure of interviewing a delightful tattoo artist from Santa Barbara, California, Pat Fish.

When Pat Fish was a child, she had no ethnic identity. As an orphan, she felt alone and yearned for a connection to a bloodline. She finally met her true Pictish, and Scottish relatives and learned of her heritage right around the time that she began tattooing, a lattice of coincidences that told her she was meant to do Celtic tattoos.

She has made many pilgrimages to Celtic lands and researched ancient illuminated manuscripts, tramped through muddy fields to see standing stones and Neolithic monuments, and spent many an hour in deserted graveyards with charcoal and paper, taking rubbings from high crosses.

Pat is a gifted artist, blessed with a kind of dyslexia that allows her to be ambidextrous and see things backwards and forwards with ease, so looking at the negative spaces and

71

interlacings in Celtic weave is something she has found to be endlessly fascinating.

In her own words: "In the past several years I have had the opportunity to meet and work with some outstanding people whose lives have been forever shaped by their encounters with the disease of breast cancer. I truly believe that the way to live a fulfilled and satisfying life is to follow what you love, and let that interior gyroscope lead you to the things that make you happy. Tattooing allows me to be an agent of completion, a person who helps others to achieve a goal of wearing art on their bodies, in their skin, that can never be taken from them. For every person, there should be passions, enthusiasms, even obsessions, that can rightly give a clue as to what the appropriate tattoo should be. It is never for me to say what image a person should choose; your body is a temple and I'm just there to paint the walls. Every woman is unique, with her own special beauty. A tattoo can celebrate this with jewelry that can never be lost or stolen. It is a wonderful life I have chosen. There have been many challenges and opportunities that I have been grateful for, fascinating clients and amazingly talented peers."

O'Grady: I think your work is absolutely beautiful.

Fish: Thanks so much for saying so.

O'Grady: Right now, I'm a tattoo virgin,

Fish: I prefer to think of you as being a blank.

O'Grady: My doctor wants me to wait a year before having any tattooing to my breasts.

Fish: That is very sensible; the doctor is the best judge of the strength of the skin tissue and of your immune system.

O'Grady: How long have you been working as a tattoo artist?

Fish: I began in 1984, after careers in journalism, illustration and market research. I wanted to do art full time, and I wanted to have close contact with the people who would be commissioning my artistic skills.

O'Grady: Do you do realistic nipple tattoos on reconstructed breasts?

Fish: No, I am not capable of that illusion. I do art, so the women I work with are looking to have their scars mitigated and transformed into something beautiful, not an approximation of their former anatomy.

O'Grady: How many tattoos have you done on women who have had breast reconstruction due to cancer?

Fish: About a dozen.

O'Grady: Is it harder to tattoo on a woman who has made the decision not to do reconstruction because she is down to the bone?

Fish: No, the tattooing process is very shallow, no deeper than the width of a dime, so the issue is the nerves and where they may be. With anyone whose anatomy has been shifted surgically, there are phantom pains and unexpected sensitivities where the nerves have regrown.

O'Grady: While a tattoo cannot eradicate a scar or the skin's texture, it does seem to hide it very effectively. Is it more challenging for you as an artist to tattoo over a scar?

Fish: The scar tissue is not as strong as normal skin, and so requires an adapted technique. If normal tattooing is done, it can chew up the skin and the ink will be forced out in the resultant scabbing. So we have specific ways of using a pointillist technique to build up the tattoo on top of the scar tissue. This way, there are fewer holes poked into the area, and it has a better chance of healing and retaining the ink.

O'Grady: Does the skin hold the ink differently due to the thickness of the scar tissue?

Fish: Not the thickness, per se, but the composition of the collagen in the tissues is very different, and regeneration of the skin is impeded, so when you place foreign material into it, the possibility is that it will over-react and try to force the irritant out. In this case, that would mean the tattoo ink would scab up with lymph and then peel away, leaving only part of it in the skin.

O'Grady: Have you seen any problems with infections or inflammation from tattooing over scars?

Fish: No, tattooing is fairly simple and, with minimal care, they heal well. An allergic reaction to the ink or suspension agents is always possible with someone with a suppressed immune system, so waiting until all medical treatments are completed is always advisable.

O'Grady: It is no secret that getting a tattoo has some degree of pain involved. In your experience of doing tattoos, do you think it's more or less painful to get a tattoo over these kinds of scars?

Fish: More painful, but worth it. For a woman to have undergone a medical course of treatment so severe, only to be left with a patchwork of scars, can make it hard for her to focus on the positive and remember that the scars represent survival. Artistic tattoos can be transformative and freeing, making beauty and camouflaging the painful memory.

O'Grady: Do you ever use any kind of numbing medication on the area to be tattooed? If so, does this have any negative effect on the final outcome of a tattoo?

Fish: I do not. I know many artists do, but in my experience, they made the skin rubbery and difficult to work with, to the point that I had to go over much of the work a second time. I think that the pain is a transformative process, and bearing it for the desired result is part of the price you pay.

O'Grady: I have always felt that women can endure more pain than men; would you agree with that?

Fish: Women tend to acknowledge that the pain is happening, and then steel themselves to endure it for the sake of the beauty to follow. In our culture, women learn young that sometimes transformative processes thought to give greater physical attractiveness require painful resignation. Men, on the other hand, have been taught not to acknowledge pain, and so will try to tough it out and so end up making it harder on themselves.

O'Grady: I feel that by producing a piece of beautiful artwork to disguise these scars, it is possible for a woman to gain the sense of reclaiming her body, and regain self-confidence. Do you notice a visible change in these women when their tattoo has been completed?

Fish: I have had phone calls from family members thanking me, telling me that the change in their loved one is remarkable. The women themselves will tell me that after having been submissive and cooperative through all the medical tortures, and having completed the course of treatment, the tattoos I have done for them are a statement that their body is once again their own. And once again a thing of beauty in their eyes.

O'Grady: I know that you truly specialize in Celtic design tattooing, and I would think the intricate patterns would work well to cover up scars.

Fish: It is actually difficult to conform Celtic design to the body, and if there are scars, it is necessary to adapt the pattern so that if there IS ink rejected by the body, it has the minimal visibility within the pattern. I do all sorts of tattooing; my particular love is Celtic and Pictish work, but I am very happy reproducing botanical prints and any precisely rendered archival material.

O'Grady: Many women want to feel as feminine as possible after losing their breasts and desire girly-girl tattoos, which usually consist of pinks and pastel colors, flowers and such. Are certain color inks better than others for this kind of scar cover-up tattoo?

Fish: Sensitivity to the different contents of tattoo inks is usually not an issue, but with someone whose immune system has undergone chemotherapy or radiation, it is possible that they might have a reaction to red pigment, which is included in pinks and purples and lavenders. If there is any question, a tattoo should be begun with only the black ink, because carbon is the most neutral. If they heal it well, then add in blues, and work up through the color spectrum. It is extremely rare for anyone to have a reaction to a tattoo if they are in good health and use proper aftercare, but with someone with a suppressed immune system, care and caution is wise.

If you would like to contact this talented artist for an appointment:

Pat Fish
Luckyfish, Inc.
2007 State Street
Santa Barbara, CA 93105
(805) 962-7552
www.luckyfish.com

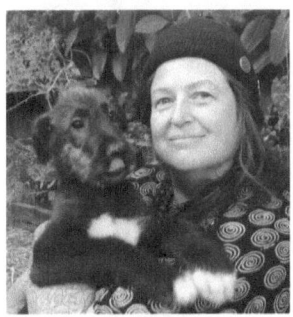

Pat Fish

The following picture features a beautiful tattoo created by Pat Fish, which she says was her greatest challenge. Her client Beth was a real trooper, and was willing to come and do many sessions to achieve this result. The butterfly is an ancient symbol for rebirth and transformation—how fitting.

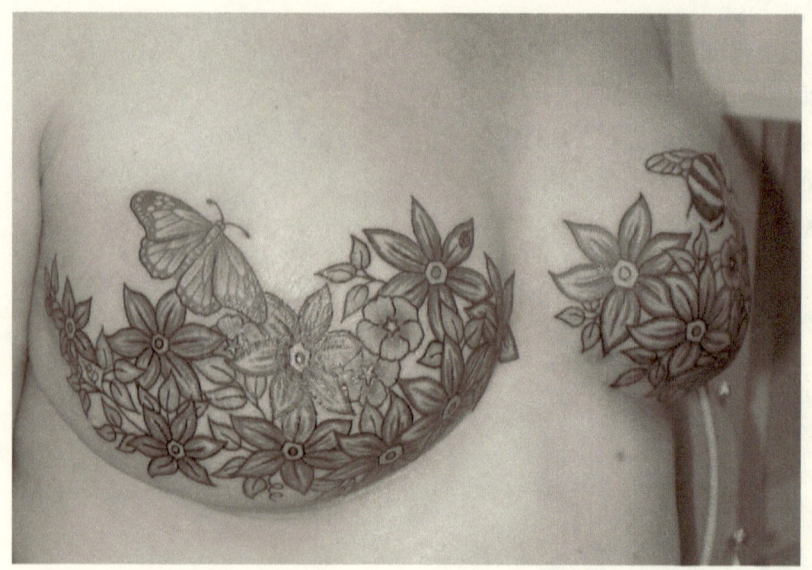

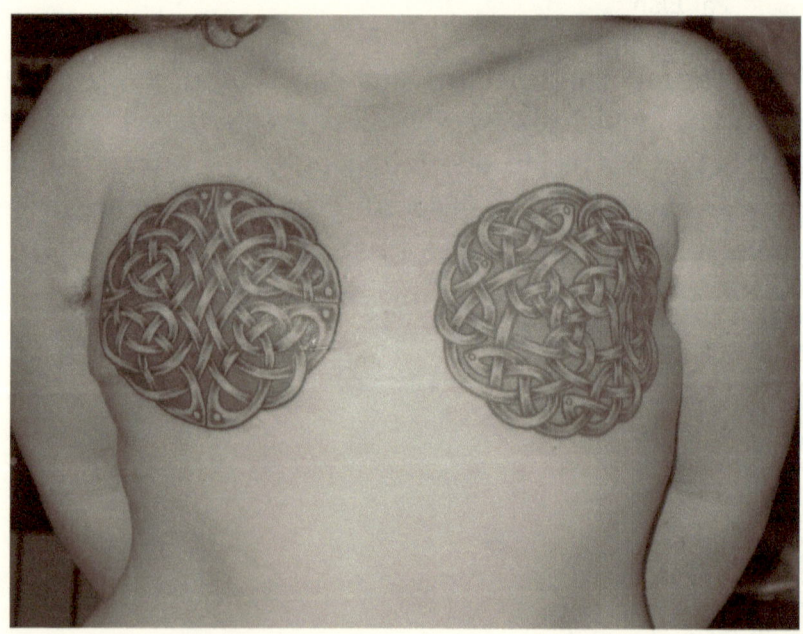

Another tattoo by Pat Fish. This gal did not opt for reconstruction and so covered the relatively flat areas with circles to represent the breasts.

# RACK WAR—Bra shopping

This might seem like an easy task, but after breast reconstruction, it can be a nightmare. Breast reconstruction can create some unique bra problems, so it's best to be mentally prepared before you even begin.

Immediately after your implant surgery, the doctor will want you to wear a bra that gives all of his hard work good support. You can start out wearing either a medical-grade compression bra or a sports bra. This will hold your breasts in place while you heal and help reduce swelling, plus it can also aid with proper drainage. You want something with a soft cup and definitely no underwire bra at the early stages.

In most cases, you will end up wearing a different size bra than you did before your reconstruction. The bra style that you wore before surgery may not be the right choice for you now. Chances are your new breasts are positioned higher on your chest and will be different in shape than your original set. We are creatures of habit, and I bet that you have probably worn the same style bra for years. When it comes to bras, I understand that change can be hard.

After I had completely healed from my implant surgery, I wanted to start to wear a real bra, and my doctor gave me the go-ahead. I was tired of wearing a sports bra, which does absolutely nothing for anyone's shape because they tend to just flatten you out. I was anxious to show off my new assets, and I hit the stores ready to dress up the girls. I needed to celebrate beating breast cancer and having reconstruction; this day was going to be about me, and I went alone so that I could take my time and not be distracted. I walked into the store with grand illusions of pretty satin and lace bras and went straight to the racks determined to find the perfect bra. I knew that my size would be different, so I grabbed several different sizes in my usual style. The first bra didn't fit, second bra didn't fit, and third bra didn't fit, and so on. It seemed that no matter what size I tried, I just couldn't get the proper fit. If the bra fit me correctly around, the cups didn't seem right; either I didn't fill out the tip of the cup or my cup runneth over, spilling out side boob. Now from a practical standpoint, it seemed logical that if I didn't fill out the cups at the tip, I needed to just go down a cup size, but that didn't seem to be the case. It didn't seem to matter what size I tried; none of them worked. I was determined and kept on trying one after another, until I had gone through about 40 bras. It reached the point where I broke into a sweat, a full-blown hot flash, and began to feel slightly nauseous. I was weak and physically exhausted from undressing and redressing, and making the trips back and forth from the racks into the dressing room, because they only allowed six garments in at one time. I actually ended up sitting down on the tiny bench in the small private dressing room, and I felt the tears welling up in my eyes from the frustration. Then I got angry at myself; was I really crying and feeling sorry for myself because I couldn't find an over-the-shoulder-boulder holder? Feeling entirely too emotional, I pulled myself together and decided today just wasn't my day. I no longer had the energy required for the job and went home defeated and perhaps a tad bit depressed.

I needed help, but on some level, I was embarrassed to ask for a professional bra fitting because I didn't have any nipples or areolas yet. I knew that was just plain silly, but I wasn't comfortable with my body yet. I convinced myself that the real problem was the fact that my breasts weren't completed yet. Once I had my nipples and areolas, I would fill out the cups and everything would be just fine, which did have a little truth to it. Bra cups are designed with extra space to fit the nipple, so the bra cup can gap or dent at the center of the reconstructed breast, but this wasn't my only problem.

I was making another very big mistake. Every bra I tried on had one common denominator: all the same style, one that I had worn for over 25 years. I was attempting to put high, full implant breasts into the same style I wore to lift my old saggy ones. Of course this wasn't going to work; what was I thinking? The shape of the bra and cup were completely different from what I now needed. When shopping for bras, you must keep in mind that implants tend to be wider than natural breasts. I was smart to try many different sizes, but I hadn't thought about trying different styles. I was stuck in my old rut of trying on what I had been used to.

If you are in the transition time of having no nipples, you can still wear a normal bra, but it has to be the right style. Look for a triangle bra that has a heavy lining. A lined or molded bra will also help make uneven breasts look more symmetrical. If you have one breast that is slightly smaller than the other (a common problem even with natural breasts), a good trick is to make that strap just slightly tighter, giving that breast just a little more lift. Most women who have reconstruction will wear a bra without an underwire at this stage. In addition to being comfortable, non-underwire bras tend to be more forgiving when one breast is larger than the other. At this stage, you can also try an add-a-size bra, which tends to be much more padded at the tip of the breast area, filling it out for you. These are made with fiber padding and some with water or gel.

Once you have your nipple and areola reconstruction, you can change bra styles. I personally recommend a half-cup push-up bra with an underwire. Reconstructed breasts seem to fill this one out nicely, and I find that this gives me a great look in clothing, which is exactly what a bra is supposed to do. Be careful that your bra isn't too tight, and that it isn't cutting into or directly over your incisions on your sides, or it will seriously irritate them. Stay away from full-cup bras because that is where you will have the most fitting issues. Reconstructed breasts have a different shape than a natural or even an augmented breast, and you will always have a tough time getting a full cup to actually fit you correctly. Besides the fitting issues, I personally think full-cup bras look like granny bras. They remind me of the old cross-your-heart bras that my mother wore back in the day, the ones that came folded in a small box.

Don't be brand loyal. Bra sizes run differently according to style and manufacturer. If you buy several different brands, don't be surprised that they can be all different sizes yet fit the same. If you have always worn a certain brand, try a few others; this is your time to experiment.

Don't be stubborn. When you are beat, accept it and ask for help. Have a bra fitting with a true professional; you have nothing unique that they haven't already seen time and again. These ladies are used to fitting women in all different stages of breast reconstruction and a good one will make you feel completely comfortable. Studies show that most women actually wear the wrong size bra anyway, and I can tell you that bra sizing can be way more difficult after reconstruction, especially if you are lacking in the patience department. All of this bra nonsense made me wonder when these devices even began to be a staple of woman's clothing.

Early bras were basically bodices designed to support the bosom. (French; brassiere). The history of bras seems to be intertwined with the status of women in society, the evolution of fashion and ever-changing beliefs regarding modesty and the female body. Women have used a variety of garments and devices to cover, restrain, reveal, or modify the appearance of their breasts.

From the 14th century onward, the undergarments of wealthier women were mainly dominated by the uncomfortable boned corset, which pushed the breasts upward but sometimes made it difficult to breathe. Women were even known to have fainting spells because their corsets were too tight, claiming that they actually were cutting off their oxygen supply.

In the early 19th century, designs began splitting the corset into a girdle like restraining device for the lower torso and an upper part suspended from the shoulder. By the late 19th century, bras replaced the corset as the most widely used means of breast support.

It wasn't until the 1930s that companies began large-scale production. Wearing a bra became the unwritten rule of standard for a woman to wear and also was viewed as somewhat of a symbol of a girls coming of age. We demand more comfort in our day; bras have replaced corsets, and Spanx have replaced the old heavy girdle. Now, greater emphasis has been placed on the fashion aspects of bras. Manufacturing women's undergarments has become a multi-billion-dollar industry. With so many options available it can be mind boggling when you go shopping.

There is a website that sells bras made just for reconstructed breasts. They are passionate about giving breast cancer survivors who have undergone breast reconstruction after mastectomy a bra that solves the numerous issues many women encounter with their new breasts.

http://braggsonline.com

I have made reference to several different styles of bras in this chapter, and I want to be clear about all of them, so I have included detailed explanations of several bra designs below. Most women seriously need to be educated about the different kinds of bras that are available and what they are designed to do for us, because we tend to stick to just what we are familiar with.

## Full cup bra

The full-cup bra covers the entire breast and is designed to give more support. This is usually worn by women with larger cups because it helps to keep the shape and fullness of the breast, with the added bonus of helping to decrease back pain.

## Half cup bra Or demi

The half-cup bra gives three-quarters coverage to the breasts. This bra has a sexy look but still offers great support. These bras are ideal for younger wearers or those that still have firm breasts or implants. They give the appearance of having more cleavage and are ideal to wear with any clothing.

## Padded bra

Padded bras are fairly self-explanatory I think, but they do vary slightly because some have different padding than others. These can offer anything from just a slight lift to the bust line to a very pushed-up effect. Some padded bras may have removable insert pads that you can change depending on how big or small you might want to appear for that day. These come with or without underwire.

## Push up bra

This is very similar to a padded bra with the exception that the padding is in a slightly different place; therefore, it will give you more lift and cleavage. A push-up bra will always have an underwire. The padding in this bra is usually made of foam which gives a more natural look and feel.

## Plunge bra

Plunge bras can help you create super cleavage. There are several different depths of plunge bras available. These are good when wearing low-cut blouses or dresses.

## Triangle bra

With the triangle bra, the fabric is cut into an obvious triangular shape. This bra has no underwire. This is similar to that of a bikini top, not having preformed cups. This can be padded or have very thin fabric, and works best for smaller breasts that require less support.

## Underwire bra

The underwire bra was specifically designed to give added support and shape. Many think of these as being elegant and sexy. Some can give a deep plunge look. The word itself, simply put, means that the bra has wire underneath the cups. They can be worn with almost anything and come in various styles and designs, plain or fancy.

## Seamless bra also known as a T-shirt bra

The seamless bra has no seams on the cups or even around the band. Seamless bras tend to give a cleaner line under tighter clothing for a smooth look.

## Minimizer bra

Just as the name implies, this bra is for someone with a large size who wants to make their breasts look smaller than they are. It also gives added support. This bra is designed to help prevent spill over and gaping and give a more flattening smoother look.

## Water, gel and add a size bra

Water and gel bras contain a small pouch of liquid gel in each of the cups. This helps to give the illusion of more cleavage and improves lift. This can sometimes add almost a whole cup size. Some add-a-size bras are made with just foam padding.

## Strapless bra

This is a bra that has no shoulder straps, designed for wearing with clothes that reveal your bare shoulders.

## Adhesive bra

This is a bra that actually adheres to the breasts, having no straps or bands at all. It actually provides little support to the breasts. It is commonly used for backless and strapless dresses. The disposable version is made of paper and used with an adhesive. The reusable type is made of silicone that can be washed. This is great to conceal the nipple area, so that you aren't giving a braless appearance.

## Bandeau bra

This is a simple band of cloth in a tube shape that is worn across the breasts, which provides very little support or shaping.

## Convertible bra

This bra has straps that may be detached and rearranged in many different ways, such as halter, T-back, cross or even strapless. Two new alternatives to regular straps are beaded straps and clear plastic bra straps.

## Front closure bra

This bra has closures like hooks-and-eyes or a plastic clip that is in the front of the bra rather than the back. These bras lie completely flat at the back under clothing.

## Racerback bra

This type has shoulder straps that come over the shoulder into a V pattern very close to the neck. This is designed for sportswear or tank tops.

## Shelf bra

This bra is a rigid band with an underwire that sits under the bust-line and pushes up while covering either none or only a very narrow strip of the breast.

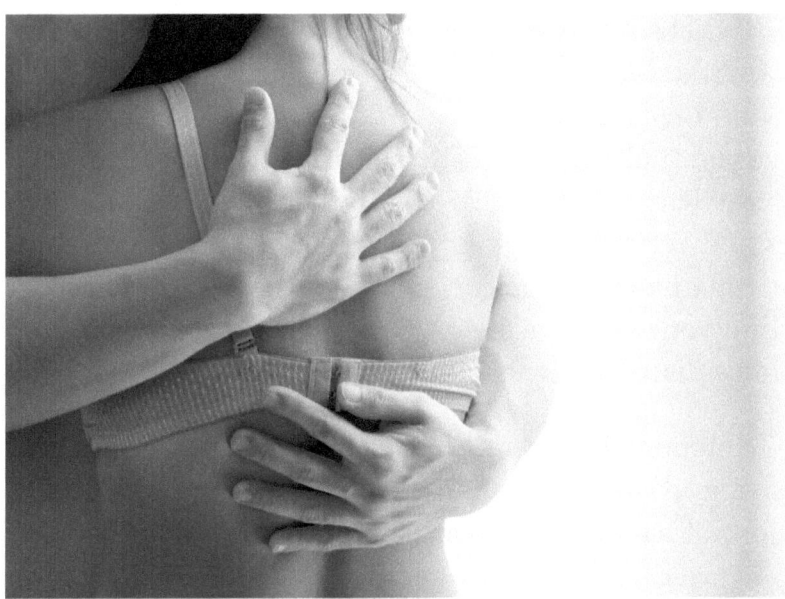

# FROM SECOND BASE TO HOME—Intimacy

You may want to know when it is safe for you to resume sexual activity. Physically, it is medically safe once you have your drains removed after the mastectomy, that is, if you desire it. Emotionally, you will most likely need more time, which is understandable. Physically, you will have days when your expanders feel extremely tight and the last thing on your mind will be having sexual relations. You may start and stop having sex during the reconstructive process several times, depending on your current stage, because obviously after each surgery you will need time to recover. You must make it clear to your partner that pressuring you is not acceptable, and that he needs to be completely supportive of you; when you are ready, you can let him know. As always, it's your body and you call the shots.

It is absolutely normal for you to have concerns about your own sexuality especially if you are less comfortable with your own body. If you have had chemotherapy, this can change your hormone levels, which can adversely affect your sex drive. If you were on any kind of hormone replacement drugs and recently stopped them, or have been placed on a hormone blocker, this can have a true physical effect on lowering your sexual drive. Any hormone balance concerns should be discussed with your doctor.

Emotionally and mentally, you may feel uneasy about not having any breasts, having expanders in your chest, having scars or not having areolas and nipples. If this is a problem, and you just don't feel sexy or attractive, try wearing a lace or satin camisole, light bra or tank top that covers that area of your body. Sexy is a state of mind; it's all in the attitude.

It is normal for you to wonder how your partner is feeling. You may worry that he no longer finds you sexually attractive. True love is not based on two mounds of fleshy fat on your chest. If he truly loves you, he will find you even more desirable. He most likely feels thankful that he didn't lose you to breast cancer, and he should have a deeper level of respect for what you are going through. He will see your strength and courage along with your beauty, and have a newfound admiration for you. If your relationship is strong, things like this should make it even stronger. You are still the same woman that he fell in love with; don't allow outside scars to change who and what you are on the inside.

Sometimes it is hard to be comfortable and confident during the process of reconstruction. While you will be looking for your partner's support, in several ways, he will also be seeking yours. It will be up to you to ease his concerns, because his problem will probably not be lack of desire for you. What is most likely on his mind is the fear that he could hurt you. In his mind, you will be fragile, and at times you must remember that you are. It will be helpful for you to be open and honest before attempting sex the first few times, and let him know what you are thinking and feeling. This way, he can reassure you that he wants you, and you can set the ground rules for what you are comfortable with. If you don't want your chest area touched, then be clear about that. Don't get discouraged if the first attempt doesn't go well; some positions will be better than others. Know that eventually all the pieces will fall into place, but until then, laugh at the confusion and live for the moment.

If you are truly having a hard time emotionally, it may help to speak with a mental health therapist or a maybe relationship counselor. Also realize that you may need to reevaluate your relationship. Respect yourself enough to walk away from anything that no longer serves you, allows you to grow or makes you comfortable and happy. At this time in your life, you need your man to really be there for you; if he has given you anything less, then you really don't need him at all, and you may be best to go it alone.

You must consider that the problem may not be with your partner but how you see yourself. You must know that your own self-worth doesn't relate to having million-dollar breasts on your chest. If you aren't being treated with love and respect, then it could be time to check your price tag. Maybe you've marked yourself down. You dictate what your worth is. Get off the clearance rack, and get behind the glass where they keep what's most valuable. If you are confident in who you are, love yourself, then and only then, can someone else truly love you.

Reconstruction recovery is not just physical; it's mental and emotional, and it is not a short process. We delight in the beauty of the butterfly, but rarely consider the changes it has gone through to achieve that beauty. You are a caterpillar soon to be a butterfly, but first you must understand that the caterpillar lives and enjoys its life during its time in transition. She may crawl on her belly, but she refuses to just stand still while she is waiting for her chance to fly. Live everyday to its fullest; don't allow the time during your reconstruction to be wasted. Enjoy yourself, always staying mindful that you do have some physical restrictions. However, don't make the mistake of using those physical restrictions as an excuse to do nothing at all.

Remember that every day gets better than the one before it. You are moving forward; don't allow yourself to go backward. In time, the scars will fade, your reconstructed breasts will become part of you, your sex life will bloom, and soon all the surgeries will become a distant memory.

# MONEY MONEY MONEY

Breast reconstruction doesn't come cheap, so how do you manage to pay for it all? After having the diagnosis of breast cancer, and then having a mastectomy, one of the last things a woman should need to be concerned about is how much all of this is going to cost her. But sadly, for many women, that is just a reality.

If you have health insurance, know that the law protects you. The Federal Women's Health and Cancer Rights Act of 1998 (commonly known as WHCRA) includes protection for women with breast cancer that choose to have breast reconstruction after a mastectomy. Under this law, it is now mandated that insurance benefits must include coverage for:

- ✓ Reconstruction of the breast on which the mastectomy was performed.

- ✓ Surgery and reconstruction of the other breast as to produce a symmetrical or balanced appearance.

- ✓ The prostheses (or breast implants)

- ✓ Physical complications at all stages of mastectomy, including lymphedema, (swelling that sometimes happens after treatment for breast cancer)

The WHCRA can be somewhat of a complex law, because there are some insurance plans that fall under exceptions. You can call the U.S. Department of Labor's toll-free number at 866-487-2365 if you have any questions or concerns. They also have a website:

**http://www.dol.gov/ebsa/Publications/whcra.html**

Naturally, you can also call your own health insurance provider directly (a phone number should be listed on your insurance card) or your state insurance commissioner's office (find that number in your local phone book under the state government section).

This law does not apply to Medicare and Medicaid, but that doesn't mean that they won't pay for breast reconstruction. Ask your doctor to request authorization from them, and see if they will approve it. If they deny you, insist on appealing their decision and fight it. Make sure that you are aggressive; don't just accept the first "no" answer from them. Both of these plans usually cover mental health care visits. If you are suffering from severe depression, having a psychiatrist recommend that you undergo breast reconstruction can be very helpful when the insurance company is making a final decision during the appeal process.

If you have *no health insurance* or you are unable to get coverage for this procedure through your insurance company (such as in the case of Medicare or Medicaid), there is still help available, so don't despair.

You may be able to get financing for breast reconstruction by applying through an organization like CareCredit, which offers payment plans for as long as 60 months. Many plastic surgeons can give you information about available options. For more information, you can go to the website at:

**http://www.carecredit.com**

There is a wonderful foundation called My Hope Chest that raises money through donations. They can offer financial help to women who have no medical insurance to cover breast reconstruction costs. If you plan to apply to this foundation for assistance, be aware that they always have a waiting list, sometimes a long one. The sooner you get on the list, the better off you will be.

This is a general outline of the criteria you must meet to be considered for the My Hope Chest Program.

Criteria:

The patient must be 69 years of age or under, free of medical complications that would preclude safe surgery (as determined by one of their participating surgeons and medical consultants), able to show demonstrable need* and a legal resident or citizen of the United States. *Demonstrable need shall include consideration of the following criteria.

1. Uninsured

2. Proof of non-eligibility for Medicaid annually

3. Income that does not support self-funding of care.

4. Hardships or exceptional circumstances

http://**www.myhopechest.org**

If you just can't stand the thought of being on a waiting list, you can do your own fundraising, with the help of family and friends. There are many options, including candy sales, bake sales, car washes and other fundraising events, so be creative. Don't forget about the Internet, which has made it very easy to raise funds for the right causes. You can use an online fundraising website to get donations. Make a profile on one or more of these sites, but make sure that you link it to your Facebook page; this will show that you are a real person and your cause is legitimate. Pages that aren't linked to an established Facebook account seem to get zero donations because they appear suspicious and phony. Most people are well aware of con artists on the Internet scamming others for money, so make sure you take your time filling out the profiles on these sites; be detailed, and including just a few pictures of yourself can be very helpful.

http://www.giveforward.com
http://www.indiegogo.com
http://www.gofundme.com
http://gogetfunding.com
http://**www.crowdrise.com**
**http://24fundraiser.com**

# THE BREAST OF TIMES—
## History of breast cancer

Breast cancer is not a new disease; it has been known to mankind since ancient times. They may not have had an official name for it, but it is clear from the descriptions of visible symptoms recorded on papyrus in ancient Egypt that the disease existed even in those days. Unlike other internal cancers, breast lumps will evidently manifest themselves as visible tumors, and the ancient Egyptians were the first to really make note of the disease.

We've come a long way, baby. The ancient Egyptian doctors would have cauterized a breast in hopes of simply burning out the disease. They didn't have mammograms, ultrasounds or MRI machines, or any real true understanding of what was happening to these women. In some cases the treatment for breast cancer was so terrifying that women often ignored any signs of their disease. If they found a lump, they hid it, and I can't say that I blame them. Their breasts would then become disfigured as the tumors just took over their bodies, but clearly they had few options, unlike today. There were no pretty pink ribbons, or encouraging chants or breast cancer walks or support groups.

Hippocrates, the father of Western medicine, spoke about breast cancer and thought it was caused by the excess of black bile, and then scientists like Galileo and Newton also had their different theories about what caused the disease.

George Washington's mother died from breast cancer as well as Queen Mary. The daughter of President John Adams, a founding father and second president of the United States, Abigail "Nabby" Adams had breast cancer. She received a mastectomy in 1811, in which she was tied to a chair, without the use of any anesthesia. Shockingly, this was a common practice in the 18ᵗʰ century. The gruesome details of her surgery have been well documented by historians. Even after enduring such a barbaric operation, her cancer continued to spread throughout her body, and she died at the young age of 48.

Luckily, in the 19ᵗʰ century, anesthesia was developed. Breast cancer surgery was then revolutionized by Dr. William Halsted. He popularized the radical mastectomy as the treatment of choice for any woman with breast cancer. Even though an extreme amount of tissue was removed, it must be noted that women were surviving the operation and their breast cancers. He removed not only the breast, but also the lymph nodes and the chest muscles. It has been recorded that in extreme cases, some surgeons performing radical mastectomies included the practice of removing part of the rib cage. This, however, proved to be so disfiguring that the practice was soon stopped. With the awakening of the women's movement, radical procedures have been examined and questioned, leading to the development of the modified mastectomy with sentinel lymph node biopsy. Before long, the art and science of breast reconstruction emerged.

The first true attempt at breast reconstruction was in 1895. Surgeon Vincent Czemy, a professor of surgery, is credited with the first autogenous breast reconstruction. He transplanted a fist-sized lipoma from the patient's flank, after he had removed her breast tumor, and the operation was a success.

There were other experiments by doctors, some with disastrous results, like paraffin injections. Physicians tried several substances for creating a breast implant, including ivory, glass balls, ground rubber, ox cartilage, Terylene wool, and polyether foam sponges.

During World War II, Dow Chemical Company created the first silicone breast implants for cosmetic breast augmentation. Other companies soon followed manufacturing implants for cosmetic augmentation and reconstruction surgeries. Women found that these silicone implants looked and felt better than the saline alternative. The early-generation devices had problems over time. Some silicone implants leaked, which caused scarring and deformities. Mass litigation followed, with claims of autoimmune diseases and cancer. The FDA banned them, and Dow Corning stopped producing implants, which put the company into Chapter 11 bankruptcy.

Between 1992 and 2006, saline-filled implants were the only approved implants on the market in the United States. Large-scale studies of the health effects of silicone were still being performed after numerous reports from the Mayo Clinic, the National Institute of Medicine and a national study, it was confirmed that silicone breast implants were not connected to other cancers or lupus. In 2006, the FDA reversed its ban on silicone-filled breast implants, stating that they had determined them to be safe and effective. These newer-generation devices are the safest, softest and most natural-looking implants to date. Women can now choose either saline or silicone implants; both are being used today.

The future is even better for breast reconstruction and breast cancer patients. It was a long, hard journey, in which many women truly suffered to pave the way for us. We have new, improved surgical procedures, anesthesia, excellent pain management drugs and higher-quality implants. Doctors have a much better understanding of how to treat a breast cancer patient as a whole, taking into consideration not only how she is doing physically, but mentally and emotionally as well. Women are beating the odds, living longer and looking better than they ever had before.

I had been under the wrong impression that breast cancer was a disease of our time, perhaps having only been around for two centuries at the most. I suspected that it was caused by pollutants and chemicals we expose ourselves to on a daily basis. The hair dyes, deodorants, cleaning products, perfumes, pesticides, processed foods, our over indulgence in all things bad like fast foods, diet colas and sugary sweets. Clearly, my thinking was wrong about this, although I'm sure that these things haven't helped our overall general health. In Cleopatra's time women would have been consuming whole grains, fish, fresh fruits and vegetables grown organically in rich soil. Their drinking water was pure as was the air they breathed, yet they still battled this disease.

According to the American Cancer Society, it is estimated that in the United States, about 232,000 new cases of invasive breast cancer are diagnosed each year. About 64,000 new cases of carcinoma in situ of the breast will be found (which is the earliest form of breast cancer). They estimate about 39,000 deaths a year are caused by breast cancer. Breast cancer is the most common cancer among women in the United States, and it is the second leading cause of cancer death in women. The chance of a woman having invasive breast cancer during her life is about 1 in 8, but the chance of dying from breast cancer is about 1 in 36. Breast cancer death rates have been steadily going down each year. This is probably the result of finding the cancer earlier; we certainly have learned that early detection saves lives. It is estimated that more than 2.8 million breast cancer SURVIVORS are in the United States alone.

We may be winning the battle, but at what point can we just stop the war? Shouldn't we be further along than we are in completely annihilating breast cancer? Where does all that money go that is collected for breast cancer research? Most of your donations are spent on education, screening, treatment and even more fundraising, and of course, administrative costs including salaries. Little is actually used for research despite the fact that some organizations say that their top priority is finding a cure. Be careful where you donate, and know what your money is going to be used for. I don't want to donate to someone's $500,000 annual salary. Maybe it's time we stopped with all the pink fluff and just got angry. I want answers. Why did I get breast cancer and, more importantly, how can I keep my daughter from getting it?

Breast cancer does not discriminate. It can hit anyone, no matter what sex or race, or how famous, glamorous or rich. You may have days when you feel completely alone, but many are walking the same path as you.

# INSPIRATION

With the completion of this book, today I close the door to the past, open the door to the future, take a deep breath, step on through and start the next chapter in my life, whatever that will be.

I always say that everything we go through in life is for a reason. We grow and change with each person that enters or exits our life. In some cases, you are destined to give, or the other person will give something to you or at its best, you'll enjoy an equal balance of both. With every trial and adventure, we evolve out of sheer necessity, and we hope that these changes make us better people, not worse. Having survived breast cancer, I can't help but feel that I have been given a new lease on life. I've always known that tomorrow is promised to no one, and that life is a precious gift, but sometimes maybe we need something to remind us of these things. This experience has truly made me appreciate the time I have been given, and I will remember that each and every day. I plan on not even wasting one second of it. We all have a purpose in our life, and you must find your own.

Sooner or later, everyone will face some crisis in their life that they cannot manage. There will come a point when the only hope you have left in this world will be a miracle. To see my own mother survive stage 4 breast cancer and still be here 33 years later to talk about it, with no cancer recurrence, only proves that miracles can and do happen. I prayed for and received my own miracle, when my hair was spared because I didn't require chemo. It may seem vain and somewhat trivial, but God knew it was important to me. We all have different coping skills; for me, the support of my friends and family, my faith in God, and the time that I spent in prayer carried me through all of this. In Christ, we find purpose for the pain, strength for the struggle and faith for the fight. Feed your faith and your fears will starve to death.

*I could see only one set of footprints.*
*So I said to the Lord, "You promised me, Lord,*
*that if I followed you, you would walk with me always.*
*"The times when you have seen only one set of footprints*
*were when I carried you."*

* 9 7 8 1 4 9 1 8 6 6 9 3 1 *